Everyday Law
for Seniors

The Everyday Law Series
Edited by Richard Delgado and Jean Stefancic
University of Pittsburgh Law School

Everyday Law for Individuals with Disabilities
Ruth Colker and Adam Milani (2005)

Everyday Law for Children
David Herring (2006)

Everyday Law for Gays and Lesbians
Anthony C. Infanti (2007)

Everyday Law for Consumers
Michael L. Rustad (2007)

Everyday Law for Latino/as
Steven W. Bender, Raquel Aldana,
Gilbert Paul Carrasco, and Joaquin G. Avila (2008)

Everyday Law for Immigrants
Victor C. Romero (2009)

Everyday Law for Seniors
Lawrence A. Frolik and Linda S. Whitton (2010)

Forthcoming
Everyday Law for Women
April Cherry

Everyday Law for Patients
Alan Scheflin and A. Steven Frankel

Everyday Law
for Seniors

Lawrence A. Frolik
and Linda S. Whitton

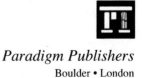

Paradigm Publishers

Boulder • London

Copyright © 2010 Paradigm Publishers

Published in the United States by Paradigm Publishers, 3360 Mitchell Lane Suite E, Boulder, CO 80301 USA.

Paradigm Publishers is the trade name of Birkenkamp & Company, LLC, Dean Birkenkamp, President and Publisher.

Library of Congress Cataloging-in-Publication Data

Frolik, Lawrence A.
    Everyday law for seniors / Lawrence A. Frolik and Linda S. Whitton.
        p. cm. — (The everyday law series)
    Includes bibliographical references and index.
    ISBN 978-1-59451-701-3 (hardcover : alk. paper)
    1. Older people—Legal status, laws, etc.—United States.   I. Whitton, Linda S.
II. Title.
    KF390.A4F7535 2009
    346.7301'3—dc22

                                    2009030848

Printed and bound in the United States of America on acid-free paper that meets the standards of the American National Standard for Permanence of Paper for Printed Library Materials.

Designed and Typeset by Mulberry Tree Enterprises.

14   13   12   11   10   1   2   3   4   5

Contents

Acknowledgments

I owe a special thanks to my research assistant, Amie E. Schaadt, Pitt Law 2007, for her efforts in the creation of this book. I also wish to thank the staff of the University of Pittsburgh School of Law Document Technology Center—Phyllis Gentille, Karen Knochel, Darleen Mocello, Barbara Salopek, and the director of the center, LuAnn Driscoll—for their assistance in the creation of the manuscript of this book.

               —Lawrence A. Frolik

I owe a debt of gratitude to my husband, Dr. John Harris, for cheerfully serving as our critical senior reader. Many thanks also to my research assistant, Meghan Beeler Pridemore, Valpo Law 2008, for the helpful Internet resources she gathered to benefit our readers.

               —Linda S. Whitton

1
Law and Seniors

Did You Know?

- Your average life expectancy at age 65 ranges between twenty and twenty-three additional years, depending on your gender.
- Twenty-five percent of those who reach age 65 will live to at least age 90.
- The percentage of the population over age 85 is continuing to increase.
- The likelihood of a person developing a chronic disabling condition or dementia increases significantly after the age of 85.
- If you retire at the normal Social Security retirement age, you may live more than twenty years without earned income.

Who Are "Seniors"?

A book about the law and seniors must necessarily define what is meant by the term "senior." Popular senior discounts are triggered at a variety of ages. For example, you can qualify for AARP membership as early as age 50, but not for a National Parks Senior Pass until age 62. The ages at which movie theaters, restaurants, and other businesses offer special senior discounts often range anywhere from age 55 to age 65.

Although chronological age is certainly one way of determining whether you qualify for senior status, it tells us very little about you as an individual. In reality, no particular chronological age can tell us much about how anyone ages. Indeed, some persons seem old at age 65, whereas others much older seem young in terms of their physical and mental abilities.

Studies confirm that individuals of the same chronological age show great differences in mental and physical abilities. Even within the same individual, physical and mental capabilities often deteriorate at different rates. When a doctor tells a 70-year-old physically fit patient that she has the heart of a 50-year-old, the doctor is focusing on the functional level of her cardiovascular system rather than its chronological age. Not only do individuals age at different rates; so do their bodies. For example, an Alzheimer's patient with severely diminished mental function may still be in sound physical condition.

Determining what senior status means is further complicated by the wide range of ages that fall under this umbrella term. For example, a 65-year-old son and his 87-year-old father may both be described as seniors and yet have very different needs. With the increasing number of individuals who are living to age 100 and beyond, a person could potentially qualify as a senior for more than thirty years!

Given the diverse population to which society applies the label "senior," why make the distinction at all? The answer is that society and the law use chronological age and senior status for practical reasons. Age-based categories are a more cost- and time-efficient way to provide special benefits than are case-by-case individual evaluations.

The use of arbitrary age requirements to trigger benefits eligibility does not, however, always yield just results. For example, federal law provides that those who are age 65 are eligible for Medicare, a federally subsidized health care insurance. Thus, at age 63, Cindy is not eligible for Medicare even though she is unemployed and in poor health, but Bob at age 66 is eligible even though he is a millionaire who has barely been sick a day in his life.

Although basing eligibility for benefits on an arbitrary age requirement may not always produce satisfactory results, experience suggests that the law often performs poorly when eligibility is based on individual case-by-case evaluations. For example, Social Security pays benefits to younger, disabled workers who can substantiate that they are unable to work. Determining who is disabled, however, is not always easy. Often individuals believe they are disabled, but the Social Security Administration disagrees and rejects their claims. The result is excessive delays in benefits to deserving claimants and a disability system clogged with numerous appeals. In contrast, Social Security old-age benefits are paid to all who have reached their full retirement age. There is almost no litigation because either the individual is age 66 (the current eligibility age) or is not. No one can argue with the date on a birth certificate.

Although chronological age—usually age 65 or older—is arbitrarily used by the law to establish eligibility for a number of senior benefits, an important underlying question remains: Why should seniors receive special treatment? The answer to this question is complex and based on a number of demographic and policy considerations.

Even though we all age in different ways and at different rates, in time most of us will suffer a decline in physical strength, flexibility, and endurance, as well as deterioration in hearing and vision. Some will experience serious physical ailments such as congestive heart failure or stroke, and others will experience a decline in mental ability ranging from short-term memory loss to serious dementia. Based on the probability that most seniors will need some degree of help as they age—assistive services, supplementary income, or access to health and long-term care benefits—they receive special treatment under the law. The remainder of this chapter outlines factors that are relevant to why seniors receive this special treatment.

Population Age Trends

The number of seniors in the United States is increasing, as is the percentage of seniors in the total U.S. population. In 2008, about 13 percent of the population was age 65 or older. The percentage of seniors will remain at about 13 percent until the "baby boomers," those born between 1946 and 1964, begin to turn age 65 in 2011. Then the percentage will gradually rise to about 20 percent sometime after 2020.

The actual number of seniors and the percentage of seniors in the total population are increasing both because of declining birthrates and because of longer life expectancies. Not only do more individuals survive until age 65; they also have a longer life expectancy once they reach that age. In 1950, the average life expectancy of a U.S. resident was 68.2 years; by 1985, that figure had increased to 74.9 years. In 2005, it was 77.7 years. More revealing, however, is the life expectancy, not at birth, but at age 65, when women can expect to live twenty-three more years and men about twenty years. In fact, of those who reach age 65, more than 25 percent will live to at least age 90.

Seniors, those age 65 or older, are a diverse population, and it may not make sense to group someone age 65 with someone age 90. In fact, gerontologists subgroup seniors into the "Young Old," those age 65 to 75; the "Old," those age 75 to 85; and the "Old Old," those age 85 and older. Although there may be differences of opinion about where the dividing lines should be drawn for these subgroups, by whatever age someone is considered old, surely those over age 85 qualify.

Today more than 4 million Americans are age 85 or older, with the number growing at an ever-increasing rate. Some are alarmed at this, noting that those over age 85 are more likely to suffer from chronic illnesses, are heavy users of medical care and long-term care, are more dependent and likely to need supportive living arrangements, and have higher levels of poverty. The current legal and social support systems for seniors were created when the number of older individuals was much lower. Some commentators fear that our current programs for assisting seniors, particularly Social Security and Medicare, will become too expensive in the years to come as the number of seniors, and particularly those age 85 and older, continues to climb.

Gender and race are also important elements in understanding the challenge of our increasingly older society. Because women outlive men, there are only seventy-four men age 65 and older for every one hundred women.

The older the population is, the greater is the gender disparity. For example, there are only forty-six men over the age of 85 for every one hundred women. The gender disparity is important because older women on average have lower incomes and fewer savings than men. The health needs of older women differ from those of men, and some would argue that older women have different social needs.

Unfortunately, for a host of economic, health care, and cultural reasons, an African American has a shorter life expectancy than a Caucasian. For example, whereas the average life expectancy of a Caucasian male age 65 is about twenty additional years, the average life expectancy of a 65-year-old African American male is only sixteen additional years. Older African Americans on average have poorer health than Caucasian Americans and suffer higher rates of poverty. Consequently, support from governmental programs—such as Medicare, which provides subsidized health care coverage, and the federal food stamp program, which fights poverty—is critically important to the well-being of many older African Americans.

Physical Effects of Aging and Health Concerns

With advanced age comes an inevitable decline in physical vigor and well-being. Bones gradually lose calcium, become weakened, and may fracture. Joints are likely to become stiff and painful, thus making everyday activities more difficult. Stairs may become an impediment and possibly even a danger. A decline in balance, physical strength, and endurance may also threaten independence. Macular degeneration, or the loss of core vision, affects millions of seniors, preventing them from driving and reading. Loss of hearing, known as presbycusis, is also common and may make it difficult for someone with this condition to talk to others, causing frustration and a sense of isolation.

The incidence of chronic conditions—permanent or long-term ailments such as diabetes, heart disease, arthritis, and congestive heart failure—rises with age, as does the severity of such conditions. Someone who lives past age 80 is very likely to suffer from a chronic condition, at least in the last few months of life. For some seniors, severe chronic conditions signal the end of life, but other elderly live for years with chronic, disabling conditions that make them dependent on others for care and assistance.

Mental decline also afflicts many, but not all, seniors. Most older persons experience mild short-term memory losses, such as trouble remembering a new phone number. Fortunately, there are simple coping strategies to deal with mild "senior moments." These include the use of lists and electronic storage of important information. For example, cell phones and computers can be programmed to store frequently used addresses and phone numbers.

Far more serious is the loss of memory caused by dementia. Most seniors do not have dementia, though the chances of developing it rise rapidly after age 85. It is estimated that from one-quarter to one-half of those age 85 or older suffer from some form of dementia. Particularly devastating is Alzheimer's disease. During the early stages, the individual suffers episodes of disorientation as to time and place. Failing memory produces confusion and uncertainty. As the disease progresses, mental and physical skills decline until the victim loses the capability of self-care. In time, speech and all meaningful awareness are lost, and the individual may fall into a coma if death does not come first.

Because elderly seniors as a whole are not as healthy as the rest of the population, they are more likely to be hospitalized and have longer hospital stays. For most Americans, the cost of health care is paid by medical insurance. Given that most medical insurance is acquired as a benefit of employment, retirement often means the loss of, or a significant reduction in, medical insurance. As a result, there is significant subsidized governmental health care assistance for seniors in the form of Medicare and Medicaid. These programs raise the issue of how much health care assistance society can afford for seniors and how to allocate it. An even more fundamental question is whether advancing age reduces an individual's moral right to medical aid. Other questions include who should make the allocation decisions, whether some lives are more valuable than others, and whether the maintenance of life is always the highest priority. Our society has not formally answered these difficult questions. As with other puzzling questions of public policy, the answers are never clearly articulated, but public programs do provide a sort of answer because they reflect society's prioritization of generational rights and obligations.

Economic Vulnerability

Because of the loss of physical and mental vigor, seniors are less likely to be employed and more likely to have lower incomes. Many are economically very vulnerable, with low incomes and little or no savings. In response, America has created programs for seniors such as Social Security and Medicare. Although these financial assistance programs are open to almost all elderly, other programs, such as Medicaid, are designed to assist poor seniors or seniors made poor because of the expense of paying for their health care needs or the cost of a nursing home.

Although these programs and others have been very successful in reducing poverty among seniors, such programs are very costly. There is constant pressure on government to reduce costs (or raise more revenue) and to require seniors to pay for more of their own care. Unfortunately, there is no easy way to reduce the cost of these programs without reducing benefits.

With the increase in the senior population and the growing strain on federal and state budgets, the national debate over how much assistance should be provided to seniors has intensified. This debate brings into question whether we can expect the same level of benefits in our old age as was enjoyed by our parents and grandparents.

At present, most seniors who need financial help do receive some assistance. Consequently, in terms of percentages, fewer seniors are officially poor than are younger persons. However, that statistic underplays poverty among seniors because many have incomes just above the poverty line. They are able to survive financially only with the income they receive from Social Security and the subsidized medical care provided by Medicare. Even though not officially poor, they are impoverished and dependent upon governmental assistance.

Notwithstanding that some seniors are poor, alone, and isolated, most are married, are not poor, and are in good health. For example, at any one time only 5 percent of seniors—about 1.5 million—live in a nursing home, and most of those live there for less than a year. Most younger seniors enjoy relatively good health, have adequate though modest incomes, and live in the community, many with a spouse or life partner. Of course, that picture changes with age. The older a person is, the more likely she or he is to be poor, to be in bad health, and to live alone. In short, generalizations about the economic state of seniors are not of much use because of the wide discrepancies in individual well-being.

Social and Family Support

Due to the infirmities of old age, many seniors need support and assistance that can range from occasional help with household chores or a ride to the grocery store to daily personal assistance with dressing and bathing. If you are old and in need of help, it is likely to be provided by your spouse, family, and friends or possibly by volunteers from your church or community.

As long as you live with your spouse or a partner, the two of you can usually care for each other as needed. For example, one of you may shop for groceries, and the other one cooks. One may pay the bills, and the other takes responsibility for keeping the two of you in touch with family and friends.

Those who live alone often replicate the advantages of having a spouse by calling on friends or relatives for help. For example, if you live alone, you may have an arrangement with a family member or a neighbor who checks on you daily and assists as needed. Perhaps a grandchild or niece will move in with you to help take care of the house and provide transportation.

If your needs are great or you have no one to help, you may have to hire professional assistance. In some communities, you may qualify for local, county, or state governmental free or low-cost assistance, such as visiting nurses or homemaker services. You might also obtain help from community volunteers or find assistance at a federally funded senior citizens center.

Most seniors obtain assistance from informal networks comprising spouses, relatives, and friends. Most elderly men are married and so find support and assistance from their wives. Because women live longer and because wives on average are four years younger than husbands, most married women can expect a period of widowhood. In fact, about 70 percent of women over age 75 are widows. Lacking a spouse, these older widows must turn to others for help.

The first choice is usually an adult child, although the tendency to rely upon a child depends upon the child's proximity, the family's cultural background, and the elderly individual's financial resources. Proximity has become an increasing problem because of a tendency for both children and parents to move from their home communities to pursue work or more attractive retirement communities. Even children who live nearby may not be of much assistance—perhaps because of work responsibilities or challenges in their own families, such as a disabled child, economic pressures, or personal health issues. Some children of divorced parents may not feel that they owe much assistance to the noncustodial parent or to a parent who remarried and had a child with a new spouse.

The number of seniors who rely upon a child for assistance has been undercut as well by other demographic and social trends. For example, the shrinking size of the family coupled with an increasing rate of life expectancy results in some parents outliving their children. Women are increasingly in the workforce and so are unable to devote as much time to caring for their parents as they might have in times past. Even though many seniors receive some assistance from friends and neighbors, typically they lack the support that formerly might have been provided by children.

If a child does help, usually the child is female. Despite the increased participation of women in the workforce, one study found that women constitute more than 70 percent of all the adult children identified by their parents as primary caregivers. Women are often the primary caregivers because of cultural practices that identify caregiving as more appropriate for women, particularly if it consists of personal care such as dressing or bathing. Also for some women, who on average have lower earnings than men, giving up a job or working only part time in order to care for an elderly parent represents less of an income sacrifice than it might for some men. Of course, as women rise in status and pay in the workforce, this is less likely to continue to be the case.

In the absence of spouses or children, seniors rely on friends, neighbors, and social organizations. The longer the elderly individual has lived in the neighborhood, the more reliance the individual will place on friends and neighbors. Just as important is the attitude of the individual. Many seniors are fiercely independent and self-reliant. They abhor turning to a stranger or government for help. Others live in a culture that expects them to turn to friends for assistance. Elderly Asian Americans, for example, are more likely to seek help from friends than from governmental support systems. Hispanic elders with no relatives to assist them are less likely than any other ethnic group to seek outside help in times of need.

Many seniors seek support and assistance from social or religious organizations. If you are a woman, you are more likely than a man to seek such help. Even though many seniors get assistance from a church, synagogue, or mosque, reliance on religiously affiliated groups declines as wealth increases. Well-to-do seniors can afford to buy assistance that is unavailable to poorer seniors, who must rely on volunteers or government-subsidized services.

Conflicting Values

Autonomy versus Protection

The legal problems of seniors are made more complicated by an inherent conflict in public policy goals. One goal is to maintain a senior's autonomy—the right to act independently and to make choices for oneself. The other goal is to protect vulnerable seniors from the harm that may result from self-neglect or abuse at the hands of others. This conflict raises profound questions that have no easy answers.

Consider the following example. Imagine that you are a poor, elderly person who is unable to purchase healthy and nutritious meals. How would you prefer that the government help you? A cash subsidy might seem ideal, but that would burden you with buying food and preparing it, something your health might not permit. Being poor, you do not own a car, and public transportation may be unreliable, or you may lack the strength to tote groceries home on a bus or on foot. Also, carrying cash exposes you to theft or fraud.

Instead of cash, should the government provide food stamps, or is that too paternalistic because it denies you the choice of whether to purchase groceries or to buy a restaurant meal? In many communities, the Meals-on-Wheels program provides home-delivered meals. This is very helpful to shut-ins and those who prefer not to leave home, and it also assures a nutritious meal. Yet it also denies the recipient any choice. Because you have no say as to the menu, you must eat what they deliver to you. The Meals-on-Wheels program thus offers protection against malnutrition, but at the expense of individual choice. The question is whether the goal of protection—assuring that you have enough nutritious food to eat—has been properly balanced against your right to autonomy and the dignity of choosing what you think is best for yourself.

As protection increases, autonomy necessarily decreases, and vice versa. A cash subsidy gives you the greatest range of autonomy, but the least amount of protection against malnutrition. After all, you might not be physically able to shop, or you might choose to buy lottery tickets rather than food. Food stamps offer more protection than cash, but greater autonomy than Meals-on-Wheels. You can decide what food to purchase rather than eating a prepared meal. However, although food stamps offer more autonomy in food choice, there is also the risk that you might choose to buy junk food rather than nutritious food. Thus, food stamps provide more autonomy than Meals-on-Wheels, but that increase in autonomy comes at the price of less protection.

In the designing of governmental programs to assist seniors, there is always the tension between efficient solutions and the right of the individual to freedom and dignity. Few would disagree that independent choice is preferable to control by others, but autonomy also means the power to make bad choices. Too often governmental aid for seniors does not strike the balance between choice and protection that is accomplished by our food stamp example—providing needed assistance, but with only modest limits on individual choice. Governments and other institutions often err on the side of protecting seniors at the expense of their right to choose for themselves. Because of the perceived vulnerability of some seniors, it is tempting to focus only on their need for protection and to overlook their equally compelling right to autonomy.

Generational Justice

Not only must society determine whether to favor autonomy or protection in meeting the needs of seniors; it must also determine how much help to give seniors in light of the public assistance that may be needed by other segments of the population. Many point out that money directed to seniors has to come from somewhere, and that usually means from the young—those under age 65. The notion of generational justice raises the question, How much do the young owe the old? What is a just allocation of governmental aid? For example, is it just to increase spending on Medicare, or should those dollars be used to improve the health care of children without health care insurance? Is it fair to raise bus rates for the young, while giving reduced or even free fares for seniors?

Whether in the form of greater federal benefits, such as Social Security or Medicare, or more assistance from state and local governments, such as property tax relief or subsidized housing, seniors benefit greatly from governmental assistance. Some question whether the government is providing too much assistance to seniors. The burden on the young to subsidize seniors, it is asserted, is becoming too great, particularly as the ratio of the old to the young increases so that there are proportionately fewer young to pay the benefits granted to the old.

Even though seniors have serious needs, the question of whether seniors are receiving too much assistance relative to other needy segments of society is a legitimate one. Of course, there is no "right" answer. It only raises the fundamental and unanswerable questions of what do the young owe to the old, what is a good society, and what is justice?

Much of the impetus for the generational justice argument comes from the sense that seniors are reasonably well off and do not deserve the amount of assistance they receive. Some note that the measurement of senior poverty looks only at their income and not at other benefits, such as subsidized medical care (Medicare), free or reduced cost public transportation, property tax rebates, subsidized housing, and even lower fees for public recreation.

A few contend that seniors receive more than their fair share because of their political power. They argue that because a high percentage of seniors vote, politicians approve benefits for seniors in order to get reelected. Proponents of this argument conclude that the elderly should give up some of their benefits either to increase assistance for younger, needier individuals or to lower taxes for the younger population.

Others argue that intragenerational injustice exists between poor seniors and more-well-to-do seniors. The two most expensive benefit programs for seniors, Social Security and Medicare, are available without regard to need. The rich and poor alike receive the same benefits. What is the fairness, some contend, of assisting well-to-do seniors while allowing other elderly individuals to remain below or only modestly above the poverty line? Instead, the argument goes, federal and state assistance programs should be based on economic need or at least poor seniors should receive more benefits relative to rich seniors. To date, this position has not gained much support.

Age Discrimination versus Justice

Although discrimination is usually thought of as a bad thing and harmful to society, that is not always the case. The dictionary definition of the word "discriminate" is the act of making or perceiving differences. In the case of age discrimination, it can be either bad or good. Most would agree that discrimination is bad when used to harm seniors, but good when used to single out seniors for assistance.

That society should condemn discrimination against seniors may be self-evident, but it is less apparent why society should condone discrimination in favor of seniors. For example, why should Medicare be available only for those who are age 65 or older and available without regard to their financial need? The simple answer is that seniors are selected as the favored group because old age, at least historically if not currently, is associated with financial need. Seniors are also perceived as a sympathetic group who deserve our assistance. Old age is seen as something to be feared because it is perceived as a lonely, depressing time of life fraught with illness and impending death. Consequently, society tries to ease the problems of old age by providing benefits to seniors.

Sympathy aside, an objective case can be made for using only chronological age as a basis for governmental assistance because it is an efficient method of identifying those who are likely in need while avoiding the demeaning aspects of need-based eligibility criteria. For example, suppose you had to prove that you were poor in order to qualify for Social Security benefits. How would you feel filling out a form that in essence declared your life a financial failure? To avoid that indignity, many programs for seniors are available to all without the need to demonstrate financial need. All are eligible and all benefit.

The counterargument to age-based benefit eligibility is that individuals ought to prepare for their old age by saving for the loss of income that accompanies retirement. Most poverty among seniors, so the argument goes, is largely the result of a personal failure to plan. The tension between these conflicting images of the deserving old person versus someone who failed to plan for the future will never be resolved, but it does underlie much of the public debate about the proper treatment of seniors.

For More Information

Administration on Aging (202-619-0724)
(http://www.aoa.gov)

Find comprehensive information from the U.S. Administration on Aging about programs and services for seniors.

AARP (202-434-AARP)
(http://www.aarp.org)

Find discussions about timely topics of interest to seniors.

DisabilityInfo.gov (800-333-4636)
(http://www.disabilityinfo.gov)

Find information about government resources for disabled individuals and their families.

Eldercare Locator (800-677-1116)
(http://www.eldercare.gov)

Find resources for seniors in any U.S. community. Links are provided to state and local area agencies on aging and community-based services.

FDA for Older People (888-463-6332)
(http://www.fda.gov/oc/seniors)

Find information for seniors on a wide range of health issues.

GovBenefits.gov (800-333-4636)
(http://www.govbenefits.gov)

Find information on more than one thousand government benefit and assistance programs.

Healthfinder
(http://www.healthfinder.gov)

Find reliable health information from the U.S. Department of Health and Human Services Office of Disease Prevention and Health Promotion.

Medicare (800-MEDICARE)
(http://www.medicare.gov)

Find information about all aspects of Medicare coverage and benefits, including enrollment, choice of plans, costs, and appeals. Links are provided to state-specific resources.

National Indian Council on Aging (NICOA) (505-292-2001)
(http://www.nicoa.org)

Find information about services and advocacy for American Indian and Alaskan Native seniors.

NIH Senior Health
(http://www.NIHSeniorHealth.gov)

Find reliable health and wellness information on a variety of medical conditions that are of particular concern to seniors.

Senior Corps (800-424-8867)
(http://www.seniorcorps.org)

Find information about volunteer programs in local communities where seniors can share their life experiences and skills. Examples include Foster Grandparents, Senior Companions, and RSVP (Retired and Senior Volunteer Program).

Social Security Administration (800-772-1213)
(http://www.ssa.gov)

Find information about retirement benefits, disability benefits, and the location of local Social Security offices. The site also includes tools for estimating benefits and deciding when to begin receiving retirement benefits.

2

Age Discrimination in Employment

Did You Know?

- If you are over age 40, you may be protected against being fired or passed over for promotion because of your age.
- Showing that you were replaced by someone younger is not enough, by itself, to prove age discrimination.
- If you are the victim of age discrimination, you should save all employer communication that reflects a negative age bias and also make note of any negative comments about age or older workers.
- Not all employment policies that adversely affect older workers more than younger workers violate the law.
- Partners, business owners, and consultants are not protected against age discrimination in employment.

Most seniors are protected against age discrimination in employment by federal law. Some are also protected by state law. If you were passed over for a job or promotion that was given to a much younger worker, or terminated from a job while other, younger workers were retained, you may have a legal claim for age discrimination in employment. The following discussion outlines what situations may give rise to a valid age discrimination claim and what situations do not.

The Age Discrimination in Employment Act

In 1967 Congress passed the Age Discrimination in Employment Act (ADEA) (29 U.S.C. §§621 *et seq.*) to protect older Americans from age discrimination in the workplace. With a few exceptions, the ADEA pro-hibits employers from discriminating against older workers with respect to hiring, firing, compensation, and conditions of employment (29 U.S.C. §623[a]). The goal of the ADEA is to promote the employment of older Americans, to ban the arbitrary firing of older workers, and to encourage employers to create age-neutral employment practices. Mandatory retire-ment on account of age, excluding a few narrow exceptions, is also prohib-ited by the ADEA. Many states have enacted anti–age discrimination statutes that are similar to the ADEA; some state statutes offer age discrim-ination protection to employees who are not protected by the ADEA.

Who Is Protected?

Not every employee is protected by the ADEA. The act applies only to in-dividuals age 40 and older (29 U.S.C. §631[a]) who work for employers that have twenty or more employees (29 U.S.C. §630[b]). The ADEA also cov-ers labor unions and employment agencies (29 U.S.C. §630). To fall within the "twenty or more employees" category of covered employment, an em-ployer must have twenty or more employees for each working day for at least twenty weeks. Thus, some part-time employees may not count in a de-termination of whether the employer meets the requirement (29 U.S.C. §630[b]). However, if the employer does fall under the ADEA, then all em-ployees, including part time, are protected.

Given that the ADEA protects only employees who are age 40 and older, younger employees may be fired or not hired because of their age. For ex-ample, suppose an employer with one hundred employees is not happy with the performance of an employee, Sarah, who is age 35. The older employees are covered by the ADEA, but 35-year-old Sarah is not protected. Her em-ployer tells Sarah, "I am firing you because you are just too young and lack the experience necessary to do your job." Sarah is not protected by the ADEA even though she was fired because of her age. The ADEA was en-acted to address age bias against older workers, not to bar age discrimina-tion against the young.

Even though the ADEA does not prohibit "reverse" age discrimination in favor of older workers (*General Dynamics Land Systems, Inc. v. Cline*, 540 U.S. 581 [2004]), it also does not require affirmative action for the ben-efit of older, protected workers. For example, it was not an ADEA violation when a university did not hire an applicant even though a hiring committee recommended that he be hired because of his age and experience (*Bryan v. East Stroudsburg Univ.*, 101 F.3d 689 [3d Cir. 1996]). If, however, an older worker is not hired or promoted and the position or promotion is given to a younger person with similar qualifications, an age discrimination claim may exist even if the younger worker is also over age 40. So long as the age difference is significant, it may be used as evidence of age discrimination by the employer (*O'Connor v. Consolidated Coin Caterers Corp.*, 517 U.S. 308 [1996]). For example, if the employer fires Laura, age 60, and replaces her with Lydia, age 44, it may have violated the ADEA.

Much ADEA litigation focuses on whether a person is an employee. The act does not protect partners, directors, business owners, consultants, or independent contractors (29 U.S.C. §630[f]; *Kennel v. Dover Garage, Inc.*, 816 F. Supp.178 [D.D.N.Y. 1993]; *Caruso v. Peat, Marwick, Mitchell & Co.*, 664 F. Supp. 144 [S.D.N.Y. 1987]). For example, Ken is a partner in a law firm that has thirty partners and eighty staff personnel. The firm has a rule that partners must retire at age 65. Because Ken is a partner, he is not protected by the ADEA, and so his firm can force him to retire. The firm, however, cannot force the nonpartners to retire at age 65 because they are protected employees.

Whether an individual is a partner or an employee turns on more than just the individual's job title. Courts look to the job description rather than the job title. If the relationship to the firm of those labeled partners is in reality one of an employee, courts will find that they are protected by the ADEA. For example, an accountant who was called a partner was found in actuality to be an employee because he had no management authority, did not participate in the firm's profits or losses, and had no ownership interest in the firm (*Simpson v. Ernst & Young*, 100 F.3d 436 [6th Cir. 1996]).

Even though a company that is subject to the ADEA cannot mandatorily retire or fire employees based on age, it is free to do so with respect to consultants and members of its board of directors. Consider the following example of Kelly, age 60, hired as a consultant by Acme Co. to provide marketing advice. If the company fires her and indicates that it did so because some of the company's officers thought she was too old to do a good job, she has no protection under the ADEA. Likewise, Acme Co. can legally require members of its board of directors to retire at age 70 (or any age) because directors are not protected by the ADEA.

Sometimes when an older individual sues under the ADEA, the alleged "employer" will claim that the individual was not an employee, but was an independent contractor and thus not protected by the ADEA. In response, the individual will argue that he or she was a protected employee. To resolve the issue, courts consider the facts and circumstances surrounding the job in question. Even if the individual was hired with the title "consultant" or "independent contractor," a court will consider the actual relationship of the individual to the employer rather than merely the title of the job. Generally, an individual will be considered an employee if the employer can dictate the time, place, and manner of employment; furnishes tools and equipment; or controls the individual's job performance (Rev. Rul. 87-41, 1987-1 C.B. 296).

Exceptions to the ADEA

Firefighters, Police, and Prison Guards

The ADEA exempts selected employees from its protection. The exemptions recognize that in some situations age may be a relevant indicator of the ability to perform job functions. Consequently, the ADEA grants government employers the right to use age as a reason to refuse to hire or to mandatorily retire police, firefighters, and prison guards (29 U.S.C. §623[j]). If the mandatory retirement policy was adopted after September 30, 1996, the age of required retirement cannot be less than age 55 (*id.*).

The exemption recognizes that if older individuals cannot adequately perform the strenuous duties required by these jobs, they might put others at risk. Absent mandatory retirement, the government would have to individually test all police, firefighters, and prison guards to see if they were fit to perform their jobs. Unfortunately, even such a test would not uncover all employees who might fail at their jobs. For example, the risk of a heart attack rises with age, but no test can reveal with certainty which employee is likely to have a heart attack. Yet if a firefighter suffers a heart attack on the job, his collapse could put fire victims or other firefighters at risk, not to mention that a firefighter who has a heart attack while on the job would be at risk of additional injury.

Executive Policymaker Exceptions

The ADEA does not protect those individuals who are employed in a bona fide executive or a high policymaking position if they are entitled to an immediate and nonforfeitable annual retirement benefit of at least $44,000 (29 U.S.C. §631[c][1]). This exception applies only to a few top-level employees and never to individuals in middle management, even if they meet the retirement income requirement. A bona fide executive is usually a manager who has the power to hire, fire, and direct the work of other employees. Whether an employee qualifies as holding a high-policy position is determined by the nature of the employee's responsibilities with respect to the direction of the company and the company's operations (*Colby v. Graniteville Co.*, 635 F. Supp. 381 [S.D.N.Y. 1986]). These are employees, such as a chief economist or chief research scientist, who lack the power of an executive but play a significant role in determining company policy.

The ADEA exclusion of high-ranking executives and policymaking individuals recognizes that companies often benefit from new leadership. Companies generally require very-high-ranking employees, such as the president or chief financial officer, to retire at a designated age. By setting a retirement age, the company avoids a debate about whether the company would be better off with new management. A designated retirement age also permits the company to plan for replacing high-ranking employees who reach the mandatory retirement age. For example, Jennifer, age 64, is president of Beta

Co., which has a mandatory retirement age of 65 for its president. Beta Co. knows that Jennifer will be retiring in one year and so can make appropriate plans to replace her.

Federal, State, and Local Government Immunity

Because of a U.S. Supreme Court decision, the ADEA does not apply to state and local governments (*Kimel v. Florida Bd. of Regents*, 528 U.S. 62 [2000]). However, state and local employees may still be protected from age discrimination under state anti–age discrimination statutes. Although federal employees are protected by the ADEA (29 U.S.C. §633[a]), specific provisions of other statutes permit mandatory retirement of selected employees such as federal air traffic controllers (5 U.S.C. §8335[a]).

Proving Illegal Discrimination

In Hiring

Only about 10 percent of ADEA complaints claim age discrimination in hiring. In most cases, individuals do not know why their employment applications were rejected and thus are unaware of any discriminatory reasons. Even if the rejected applicant has reason to believe that employment was denied because of age discrimination, proving discrimination in hiring is not easy. It is never enough to show only that a younger applicant was hired. Rather, the rejected applicant must prove that his or her age was the main reason for the employer's decision not to hire. This is very difficult to prove, though sometimes it can be shown. For example, an employer was held to have engaged in age discrimination when an applicant for a federal job was told during the hiring process, "You old timer, you've been around here. You know what this is all about" (*Lucas v. Paige*, 435 F. Supp. 2d 165 [D.D.C. 2006]).

In Termination of Employment

Most complaints filed under the ADEA arise when an employee who was fired claims that the firing took place because of his or her age. Naturally, the employer will not have announced that the employee is being fired because he or she is "too old." However, if the employee believes that whatever the employer's stated reason, the real reason for termination was age, the employee will have the burden of proving that claim.

An illegal termination because of age can be proved in any of three ways. First, the discharged employee may provide direct proof of discrimination, such as an internal employer memo, if such evidence exists. Second, age discrimination can be shown through circumstantial evidence, such as statements that show an age prejudice on the part of the employer. And third, the discharged employee may demonstrate an ADEA violation through the use of employment statistics that show a "disparate impact" on older employees—

that is, the statistics must show that the employer's policies and practices are not age neutral; they produce a greater negative effect on older employees than on younger ones. The following is an overview of each of these methods for proving age discrimination in the termination of employment.

Direct Proof. Direct proof of age discrimination requires offering explicit evidence that age was the motivation for the termination. For example, the employer may have created a paper trail such as an internal letter or memorandum to the human resources department. The memo might be employee specific — "We need to fire Smith because he is over the hill. Hire someone younger with some energy." — or it might relate to all employees over a certain age — "Terminate all marginal employees age 55 or older in order to reduce operating costs." Even a metaphorical statement about age as a reason for termination might be sufficient. In one case, a statement by a supervisor that it was necessary to cut down "old, big trees so the little trees underneath can grow" qualified as direct evidence of age discrimination (*Wichmann v. Bd. of Trustees of S. Ill. Univ.*, 180 F.3d 791, 801 [7th Cir. 1999]). An admission that age was one of several factors used to determine which employees would be terminated was also held to be direct evidence of illegal age discrimination (*Febres v. Challenger Caribbean Corp.*, 214 F.3d 57 [1st Cir. 2000]).

Because today most employers are better educated about age discrimination, few create documents like those just described. Usually, an employee who believes that he or she was a victim of age discrimination must find another way to prove the case. One alternative way to directly demonstrate illegal age discrimination is by producing evidence of an employer's negative remarks about old age and older employees. It is not necessary that such remarks were made specifically about the discharged employee. These statements are offered to prove that the employer had a bias against older workers and that this bias accounted for why the employee was fired.

An employer's remarks are considered relevant if they were age related, made in the same general time period as the termination by an individual with authority over the employment decision in question, and related to the employee's termination (*Cooley v. Carmike Cinemas, Inc.*, 25 F.3d 1325 [6th Cir. 1994]). Statements that an office needed to get rid of "old heads" and that "younger employees were running circles around the older employees" were found to be evidence of age discrimination in the termination of an employee even though the statements were not made to him at the time of his termination (*Denesha v. Farmers Ins. Exch.*, 161 F.3d 491, 498 [5th Cir. 1999]).

Circumstantial Evidence. Because most employers are careful not to leave a paper trial or to make age disparaging comments, a claimant is also permitted to prove age discrimination through circumstantial evidence. Known as a "prima facie" case, this method applies the ruling of the *McDonnell Douglas* case (*McDonnell Douglas Corp. v. Green*, 411 U.S. 792 [1973]). To prove a prima facie case, the claimant must first show that (1) he or she is age 40 or over, applied for or was employed in a job that he or she was qualified for, and was rejected despite those qualifications; and (2) after the rejection, the position remained open and the employer sought applications from persons with similar qualifications or hired a younger individual for the position who had comparable qualifications (*id.*). The younger person need not be below age 40. An ADEA violation can occur, for example, if a 60-year-old is replaced by a 45-year-old (*O'Connor v. Consolidated Coin Caterers Corp.*, 517 U.S. 308 [1996]).

If a claimant can show all the necessary circumstantial elements, the employer will typically offer alternative nondiscriminatory reasons for the dismissal, such as claiming the discharged employee was not performing well enough. If the employer is able to successfully prove a nondiscriminatory reason for the discharge, the employer will win the lawsuit. Therefore, in response to the employer's arguments, the claimant must argue that the reasons offered by the employer were merely a pretext to cover the true reason for the discharge, which was the claimant's age.

In order to successfully rebut the employer's nondiscriminatory reasons for the discharge, the claimant will have to offer proof that the employer's reasons were not the real motivating reasons for the discharge or that the reasons given, such as poor performance, were not true. Typically, the claimant will offer proof that the alleged reasons were implausible, inconsistent, or not supported by the evidence (*Brewer v. Quaker State Oil Ref. Corp.*, 72 F.3d 326 [3d Cir. 1995]). It will not be enough for the claimant to show that the reasons were bad business decisions. The ADEA is not meant to interfere with nondiscriminatory business decisions, even when the employer's business practices are unwise or the managers are mistaken about the ability of the terminated employee.

If the claimant produces enough evidence that the employer's reasons were a mere pretext for the termination, the court can find that the employer violated the ADEA (*Reeves v. Sanderson Plumbing Products, Inc.*, 530 U.S. 133 [2000]). Courts, however, are increasingly less likely to reject an employer's reasons for the discharge despite stray age-related remarks by company officials. For example, a claim of age discrimination was dismissed when the evidence indicated that the claimant's job performance was substandard despite the employer referring to the claimant as an "old man" (*Trahant v. Royal Indemnity Co.*, 121 F.3d 1094 [7th Cir. 1997]).

Winning a prima facie case is not easy. There are many reported cases in which the employee alleges that the reasons given for his or her termination were a mere pretext and that age discrimination was the real reason. Very few of these claims succeed at trial. Without direct proof of discrimination or a statistical showing of a pattern of age discrimination, most employees lose their claim for illegal age discrimination.

Statistical Pattern of Disparate Impact. The third method for proving age discrimination is by the use of statistics to show that the employer's behavior had a "disparate" (much greater) impact on older employees (*Smith v. City of Jackson, Miss.*, 544 U.S. 228 [2005]). The claimant must identify the specific employer practice or policy being challenged, show that it had a disproportionate impact on older workers, and prove that the practice caused the harm to the older, protected employees. To win a claim based on statistical evidence, the claimant must also prove that he or she was replaced by a younger worker. In response, the employer must either discredit the statistics or concede the statistics and offer a legitimate business reason for the use of a policy that disproportionately affects older workers.

Employer Defenses

There are certain lawful reasons for adverse employment decisions that can serve as employer defenses to an ADEA action. These include terminations that are part of a reduction in force, situations where reasonable factors other than age exist for the termination, jobs for which an employee's chronological age is considered a bona fide qualification, and circumstances in which the employer learns after the termination that legitimate grounds existed for the termination apart from the employee's age.

Reduction in Force
An employer may reduce its workforce in order to terminate surplus employees. When reducing the workforce, many employers terminate the highest-paid employees, who are usually the older employees. Most courts have held that it is not a violation of the ADEA to reduce the workforce by terminating only the higher-paid employees provided their positions are terminated along with the employees (*Bilas v. Greyhound Lines, Inc.*, 59 F.3d 759 [8th Cir. 1995]). For example, Acme Co. needs to cut its payroll expense by 25 percent. Rather than firing 25 percent of its employees, however, it decides to fire 15 percent of the highest-paid workers, who collectively account for 25 percent of Acme's payroll expense. Of the 15 percent fired, all but one were age 40 or older and thus protected by the ADEA. Acme Co. has not violated the ADEA. It did not fire anyone because of age, but because of high salary, and it did not replace ADEA-protected workers with younger employees.

Reasonable Factors Other Than Age Defense
When an employer fires an ADEA protected worker, the employer must be prepared to offer an explanation other than the worker's age. Almost any

reason is acceptable if the practice or policy is age neutral (*E.E.O.C. v. Johnson & Higgin, Inc.*, 887 F. Supp. 682 [S.D.N.Y. 1995]). Lawful reasons for termination include inability to perform the job, personality conflicts, insubordination, absenteeism, uncooperativeness, and low quality of production. Termination of an employee for a legally valid reason is known as the "reasonable factors other than age" defense, or RFOA. Termination may even be based on factors that are often associated with advancing age, such as an inability to work as fast or carry heavy objects, provided the termination was not based merely on chronological age.

Bona Fide Occupational Qualification Exception

Employers can also discriminate against older employees if only a younger employee is generally capable of performing the job. This is known as the bona fide occupational qualification exception, or BFOQ. This exception is limited to a few cases of physically demanding jobs or jobs that involve public safety, such as airplane pilots. The Federal Aviation Administration's regulation prohibiting commercial airline pilots from flying after age 60 was approved as a BFOQ in the 1980s (*E.E.O.C. v. Boeing Co.*, 843 F.2d 1213 [9th Cir. 1988]). Congress recently raised the mandatory retirement age to 65 (Fair Treatment for Experienced Pilots Act, 49 U.S.C. §40101).

The BFOQ exception is very narrow, and for it to apply, the employer must show that there is a sound factual basis for believing that all or nearly all persons over the age limit would be unable to perform the job or that it would be impractical or impossible to individually test such persons to see if they are qualified for the job. An employee may challenge a BFOQ defense by arguing that the employer should have relied on individual testing to evaluate job performance rather than using an arbitrary age as the reason for terminating or not hiring an older employee.

After-Acquired Evidence of Wrongdoing

If an employer violates the ADEA by firing an employee because of age, but later finds there were independent, legal reasons for termination that would have justified it, such as employee misconduct, the employer will not be liable to the employee. However, the employer must prove that the employee's misconduct was severe enough to warrant termination. For example, suppose that Beta Inc. fired Jessica, age 67, and replaced her with Ashley, age 37, for the express reason that Jessica is "too old." Jessica sues under the ADEA. Just before the trial, Beta learns that Jessica, while an employee, stole a computer worth $2,000 from Beta. In light of Jessica's theft, Beta would have been justified in firing her. Thus, although Jessica can show that Beta violated the ADEA, Beta does not have to rehire her or pay her money damages because Beta would have been justified in firing Jessica once it learned of the theft.

Enforcement of the ADEA

If you believe that your rights under the ADEA have been violated, either because you were not hired, were not promoted, were demoted, did not receive a pay raise, or were fired because of your age, you can sue your employer. Before a lawsuit may be filed, however, the law requires that you exhaust all other remedies (29 U.S.C. §626[d]). If the state in which you live has a law that prohibits age discrimination, and many do, you must first file a complaint with the proper state agency (29 U.S.C. §633[b]). Within 300 days of that filing, you must also file a complaint with the federal Equal Employment Opportunity Commission (EEOC) (29 U.S.C. §626[d]). If the state where you live has no law prohibiting age discrimination, you must file a complaint with the EEOC within 180 days of the alleged discrimination (29 U.S.C. §633[b]). After that filing, you must wait 60 days before filing a private lawsuit. If the EEOC brings a lawsuit based on your complaint, you may not initiate a private suit. You cannot sue in federal court until after you have received notice from the EEOC that it has terminated its proceedings (29 U.S.C. §626[e]). If the EEOC has not sued after 60 days, you may file suit. In the event that the EEOC later sues, your lawsuit may nevertheless continue (see generally 29 U.S.C. §626). If you are seeking unpaid wages or other monetary damages, you may request a jury trial; many claimants do so because they believe a jury will be more sympathetic than a judge (Fair Labor Standards Act §16, 29 U.S.C. §§201 *et seq.*).

Voluntary Early Retirement Plans

With the elimination of mandatory retirement, many employers rely on incentives to encourage voluntary retirement. Employer-provided benefits that serve as an incentive to retire are lawful if the employee retirements are genuinely voluntary and if the benefits are offered in a nondiscriminatory manner (29 U.S.C. §623[f][2][B][ii]). Offering a bonus of $20,000 to all workers who voluntarily retire in the next sixty days is legal. However, an early retirement plan may violate the ADEA if it favors younger employees. For example, a plan that gives early retirement benefits for each year that an employee worked for the company but grants fewer benefits for each year after twenty-five years of work is illegal.

Employers may also legally offer employees a choice of a voluntary retirement plan with extra benefits as an alternative to possible involuntary termination (*Vega v. Kodak Caribbean, Ltd.*, 3 F.3d 476 [1st Cir. 1993]). For example, the employer could announce a planned 10 percent reduction in the number of employees and provide that if enough employees volunteer to retire early, with a 20 percent increase in their retirement benefits, no one will be fired. Given such a choice, many older employees may decide it is safer to retire with the 20 percent bonus rather than risk being fired.

The employer can also require employees who select the voluntary retirement plan to sign a waiver of rights that releases the employer from liability under the ADEA (29 U.S.C. §626[f][1]). Even if the employee chooses the voluntary retirement plan, the employer may have violated the ADEA if the employee was not given adequate time and opportunity to decide whether to accept the offer. Under the ADEA, a waiver is only valid if the employee was advised in writing to consult a lawyer, given twenty-one days to consider the agreement, and given seven days after signing to revoke the agreement. Furthermore, the waiver must clearly state the rights and claims being waived by the employee. It must have been signed voluntarily and with knowledge of the rights (*id.*). Duress or mistake will make the waiver ineffective.

Older Workers Benefit Protection Act

Employers sometimes find that the cost of employee benefits, such as health care insurance, is much higher for older employees than for younger employees. The Older Workers Benefit Protection Act amended the ADEA so that an employer cannot use the existence or cost of an employee benefit plan as a justification for failing to hire or for involuntarily retiring older workers (29 U.S.C. §623[f][2]). Employers may not refuse to hire older employees in an attempt to reduce their employee benefits cost, and an employer cannot selectively reduce or terminate employee fringe benefits because of the employee's age. However, the employer can legally spend the same amount on benefits for each worker even if that amount buys fewer benefits for the older workers.

Remedies

A number of remedies are available to the employee who successfully proves an age discrimination case, including injunctive and monetary relief (29 U.S.C. §626[b]). Injunctive relief is in the form of a court order that requires the employer to do something, such as reinstate the employee, or to refrain from doing something, such as not continuing the discriminatory practice. For example, the injunction might prohibit an employer from firing the older employee.

A winning claimant can ask for reinstatement (or to be hired) (*Philipp v. ANR Freight Sys.*, 61 F.3d 669 [8th Cir. 1995]), which is the judicially preferred remedy over the granting of front pay—damages for the loss of future pay (*Woodhouse v. Magnolia Hosp.*, 92 F.3d 248 [5th Cir. 1996]). Employees who were fired are entitled to back pay from the time they were fired, and that can include loss of pay, overtime, sick leave, vacation pay, pension benefits, and other fringe benefits lost because of the age discrimination (*E.E.O.C. v. Kentucky State Police Dep't.*, 80 F.3d 1086 [6th Cir. 1996]).

A successful claimant is usually awarded attorney's fees (29 U.S.C. §§216[b], 626[b]). If the employer's violation was willful, liquidated damages equal to double the amount of the claimant's losses are awarded. An employee has a duty to lessen his or her damages (called mitigation) by seeking other employment, including the duty to accept a reasonable offer for reinstatement from the employer. Both front pay and back pay awards must be reduced by the amount the claimant could have earned using reasonable efforts during the time period in question (*Cassino v. Reichhold Chems., Inc.,* 817 F.2d 1338 [9th Cir. 1987]). The burden is on the employer to prove that an employee did not take reasonable steps to lessen damages (*Coleman v. Omaha,* 714 F.2d 804 [8th Cir. 1983]). All damages awarded under the ADEA, including back pay and liquidated damages, are considered to be a part of the claimant's federal gross income and as such are taxable (I.R.C. §104[a]; *Comm. of Internal Revenue v. Schleier,* 515 U.S. 323 [1995] [interpreting I.R.C. §104[a]]).

For More Information

Equal Employment Opportunity Commission (EEOC) (800-669-4000) (http://www.eeoc.gov)

Find information about how to file an age discrimination charge and where to find the closest EEOC field office.

3
Social Security and Supplemental Security Income

Did You Know?

- Social Security is the only source of retirement income for nearly one-half of all retirees.
- Social Security benefits are based on your work record and age (or on your relationship to a qualified Social Security beneficiary).
- A portion of your Social Security benefits may be taxed depending on the amount of your other income.
- If you are divorced, you may be entitled to Social Security benefits based on your ex-spouse's work record.
- If you are a senior with limited income and resources, you may be entitled to Supplemental Security Income even if you do not qualify for Social Security benefits.

When Social Security was created, it was intended to be one leg of a "three-legged stool" for income security in retirement, with pensions and personal savings forming the other two legs. However, today nearly three out of five retirees receive at least one-half of their retirement income from Social Security. For almost one-half of all retirees, it is their only source of income.

You must earn eligibility for Social Security retirement benefits through wage taxes paid while you are employed. Family members of workers with qualifying employment records may also be entitled to derivative and survivors benefits. In addition to retirement benefits, the Social Security Administration (SSA) oversees benefits for disabled workers and their families.

Disability benefits, like retirement benefits, are based on the disabled worker's employment record.

The official name for Social Security retirement and disability benefits is Old-Age, Survivors, and Disability Insurance, or OASDI. Although there is an "earned" aspect to both retirement and disability benefits under OASDI, there is a third type of government income benefit—known as Supplemental Security Income (SSI)—that is based not on work record, but on the recipient's status as poor and either aged, blind, or disabled. This chapter provides a general overview of the qualifications for retirement, disability, and SSI benefits. The Social Security regulations are quite complex. If you have questions about your individual entitlements, you should consult your local Social Security Administration office.

Social Security Eligibility

Only employment that is subject to wage taxes under the Federal Insurance Contributions Act (FICA) (26 U.S.C. §§3101 *et seq.*) qualifies as covered employment for Social Security purposes. An application for retirement, survivors, or disability benefits must be based on a work record during which FICA taxes were paid for the required number of "covered quarters." The required number of quarters differs depending on the type of benefit claimed. The following discussion explains FICA taxes, what constitutes a quarter of coverage, and what it means to have insured status for retirement, survivors, and disability benefits.

FICA Wage Taxes

Social Security benefits are available to workers who have paid FICA wage taxes for the required number of covered quarters of employment. Today, almost all workers, regardless of the form of employment, participate in the program. Employees must pay a 6.20 percent wage tax on earnings up to a maximum amount, which is adjusted annually for inflation ($106,800 in 2010) (26 U.S.C. §3101[a]). Employers also pay a 6.20 percent FICA tax on the employee's wages, but the employer-provided portion of the FICA tax is not considered taxable income to the employee (26 U.S.C. §3111[a]).

Whereas employees and employers share the responsibility for paying the FICA tax, self-employed individuals must pay the entire amount. To equalize the tax impact of this difference, self-employed individuals are permitted to deduct from taxable income one-half of the amount they pay in FICA taxes. Self-employment earnings of less than $400 per year are not subject to the FICA tax.

Quarters of Coverage

A quarter of coverage is the basic unit for determining whether a worker is insured (42 U.S.C. §413).[1] Although a quarter of coverage is based on a calendar quarter of three months, in actuality income need not be earned in a specific calendar quarter to satisfy the requirement. An employee's quarters of coverage for the year are computed by dividing the worker's yearly before-tax earnings by the minimum required earnings amount per quarter ($1,120 in 2010). Fringe benefits are usually not included in calculating earnings.

Even if you earn well over the minimum, you cannot receive credit for more than four quarters of coverage in any calendar year. If, however, you earn under the minimum, you can receive credit only for whole quarters. For example, consider Susan, who works only during the summer months. She earns $4,000 for the summer. Her yearly earnings of $4,000 divided by $1,120 equals 3.6 credits. Her quarters of coverage will be rounded down to the next whole number, which in this example is 3. If Susan has another job, the earnings from that job can be added to her summer earnings for the purpose of calculating her quarters of coverage.

Only wages and salaries earned in "covered employment" count toward quarters of coverage. Even independent contractors are generally subject to Social Security tax as self-employed persons. However, a few jobs are not covered by Social Security, such as federal government workers who were hired before January 1, 1984, some state and local government workers, railroad workers who are covered under the Railroad Retirement Act, most students who work for their school or college, and children under the age of 18 who are employed by their parents or who perform domestic services.

Insured Status

The number of quarters of coverage determines if a person has reached insured status and is eligible for benefits (42 U.S.C. §414). Insured status is computed based on the record of wages or self-employment income that the SSA maintains. A Personal Earnings and Benefit Estimate Statement can be requested from the SSA to determine how many quarters a person has completed. If the form contains omissions, generally tax returns and wage reports on Form W-2 can be used to supply missing earnings figures. There is an assumption that an earnings record is correct after the passage of three years, three months, and fifteen days.

Fully Insured Status. The maximum number of quarters of coverage required for any type of Social Security benefit is forty (42 U.S.C. §414[a][2]). If you have accumulated forty quarters of coverage, you are considered permanently and fully insured.

Currently Insured Status. You can claim benefits as the mother or father of a deceased worker's child if the deceased was "currently insured," meaning that the worker was credited with quarters of coverage in at least six of the previous thirteen quarters, including the quarter in which death occurred (42 U.S.C. §414[b]). Other qualifications apply to this benefit, including

- you were married to the worker,
- you have remained unmarried since the worker's death, and
- the child must be under age 16 or disabled.

Disability Insured Status. To be eligible for disability benefits, you must have worked twenty quarters out of the previous forty-quarter period, which includes the quarter in which you become disabled. Or if you became disabled before age 31, an alternative calculation requires one quarter of coverage for every two calendar quarters between age 21 and the onset of the disability. If the period of time is less than twelve quarters, then you must have at least six quarters of credit. No quarters of coverage are required to receive benefits on the basis of blindness (42 U.S.C. §423[c]).

Worker's Retirement Benefits

If you have forty quarters of coverage, you are entitled to a monthly benefit when you reach early or full retirement age. Full retirement age—also called normal retirement age—is based solely on your year of birth and has nothing to do with retirement (42 U.S.C. §416[l]). If you were born before 1938, your full retirement age is 65. If you were born after 1959, your full retirement age is 67. See Table 3.1 for full retirement ages for the intervening years.[2] Once you reach full retirement age, you can collect your full Social Security retirement benefits even if you are still employed.

Early and Deferred Retirement Options

You can choose to begin receiving retirement benefits as early as age 62 (42 U.S.C. §416[l][2]), but at the cost of reduced monthly benefits for life (42

Table 3.1   Full Retirement Age by Year of Birth

Year of Birth	Full Retirement Age
1938	65 years and 2 months
1939	65 years and 4 months
1940	65 years and 6 months
1941	65 years and 8 months
1942	65 years and 10 months
1943–1954	66 years
1955	66 years and 2 months
1956	66 years and 4 months
1957	66 years and 6 months
1958	66 years and 8 months
1959	66 years and 10 months
After 1959	67 years

U.S.C. §402[q]). Because taking benefits early means potentially more monthly benefit payments than if you waited until your full retirement age, the benefit amount is reduced proportionately. Thus, if you live what Social Security calculates to be an average life expectancy, the total benefits you receive will be the same whether you began receiving the lesser monthly amount at age 62 or the larger benefit at your normal retirement age.

If you defer receipt of Social Security benefits beyond your full retirement age, you will get a bonus in the form of higher monthly benefits to compensate for the shorter payout term (42 U.S.C. §402[w]). The amount that delayed retirement will increase your monthly benefit is based on your year of birth (see Table 3.2).

The annual increases apply for each year that you delay taking retirement benefits, up until age 70. After that point, further delay produces no further increase in benefit amounts.

The Primary Insurance Amount

The Primary Insurance Amount (PIA) is the monthly benefit paid by Social Security to a retired or disabled worker (42 U.S.C. §415). It is calculated using the average monthly earnings of the covered person while working, with inflation taken into account (called the Average Indexed Monthly Earnings, or AIME). Only wages subject to Social Security taxes are used in this calculation. For example, wages subject to FICA tax in 2010 were capped at $106,800. Any earnings above this amount are disregarded for purposes of calculating AIME.

The AIME is calculated on a thirty-five-year work record even if a person does not have thirty-five years of earnings. If, for example, an individual worked for only twenty-eight years, total earnings are still divided by thirty-five years to find the AIME. Thus, individuals who work less than thirty-five years have a significantly lower AIME than their actual average wage. For workers with more than thirty-five years of earnings, only the thirty-five years of highest earnings are considered.

Table 3.2   Delayed Retirement Benefit Credit by Year of Birth

Year of Birth	Percentage Increase for Each Year of Delay
1931–1932	5
1933–1934	5.5
1935–1936	6
1937–1938	6.5
1939–1940	7
1941–1942	7.5
After 1942	8

Although the formula results in a higher PIA for higher-income workers, it is also designed to provide a proportionately higher percentage of replacement income for lower-income workers. Lower-income retirees have about 40 percent of their wages replaced by Social Security benefits, whereas higher-income workers receive approximately 25 percent replacement of those wages that were subject to the FICA wage tax. The PIA formula is intended to be redistributive; higher-income workers' wage taxes actually pay for part of the benefits enjoyed by lower-income workers.

Derivative Benefits

Social Security benefits can be paid simultaneously to a retiree, the retiree's current spouse, the retiree's ex-spouse in some situations, and the retiree's qualified children. Benefits paid to individuals other than the retiree do not affect the amount paid to the retiree. The following explains eligibility for derivative benefits.

Spousal Benefits

Current Spouse. If you are a spouse of a retired worker, you are entitled to receive the greater of either the benefit based on your own earnings record or a benefit equal to one-half of your spouse's benefit (42 U.S.C. §402[b]-[c]). For example, Adam, age 66, is retired and receives $1,600 a month from Social Security. His wife, Alice, age 66, would receive $500 a month based on her earnings record. Instead, she receives $800 a month, or one-half of what her husband, Adam, receives. Social Security automatically pays a spouse the higher amount.

To be eligible for spousal benefits, you must have been married to the insured worker for at least one year and be at least 62 years old or have in your care a child of the insured worker who is under age 16 or who is disabled. You may receive spousal benefits only if the worker is receiving retirement benefits. Even an invalid marriage can be the basis for spousal benefits if under the Social Security regulations it is "deemed valid." For a marriage to be deemed valid, you must establish that you entered into the marriage in good faith.

If you elect to take spousal benefits before reaching full retirement age, you will receive a permanently reduced amount. However, if the insured worker collects benefits early, the reduction in the worker's benefits will not affect your derivative benefits. Likewise, if the insured worker delays receipt of benefits and is entitled to delayed retirement credits, those credits will not be included in your derivative benefits.

Consider the example of Eve, who took reduced Social Security benefits at age 62 (her full retirement age was 65). Her husband, Eli, claimed his spousal benefits at age 66, his full retirement age. Although Eve only receives $1,000 a month, Eli receives $570 a month, or one-half of $1,140, the monthly amount Eve would have received had she waited to claim benefits at her full retirement age of 65.

Divorced Spouse. If you are divorced, you may be entitled to a monthly benefit equal to one-half of your ex-spouse's monthly benefit (or a reduced portion of this amount if you claim the benefit before your full retirement age) (42 U.S.C. §402[b]-[c]). You are eligible if you are at least 62, the marriage lasted a minimum of ten years, the divorce has been final for at least two years, you are unmarried, and you are not entitled to a larger benefit on your own earnings record. Unlike a spouse, a divorced spouse can receive Social Security benefits even though the worker from whom the benefit is derived has not begun to receive benefits. Receipt of benefits by a divorced spouse does not affect the right of the ex-spouse's current spouse to also claim benefits based on the worker's record.

If you are divorced and your ex-spouse has died, you may be entitled to a benefit equal to your ex-spouse's full retirement benefit if you are at your full retirement age or are disabled and age 50 or older. The full benefit is also available at any age if you are caring for the deceased worker's child who is younger than 16 or disabled (42 U.S.C. §402[g]). You may also choose to begin receiving permanently reduced benefits as early as age 60.

Widows and Widowers. When retirees die, their spouses are eligible for an amount equal to the greater of their own benefit based on their own earnings record or 100 percent of the deceased worker's benefit (42 U.S.C. §402[e]-[f]). For example, Carlos, age 70, receives $1,000 a month in retiree benefits. His spouse, Rosa, receives $700 a month. After Carlos dies, Rosa will receive $1,000 a month. If the retiree had chosen an early retirement, the spouse would receive 100 percent of the reduced amount. If the surviving spouse has not yet reached full retirement age, the benefits are reduced based on the number of months left until full retirement age.

A surviving spouse is eligible for survivor benefits starting as early as age 60 (or age 50 if the surviving spouse is totally disabled). Surviving spouse benefits are payable only if the surviving spouse was married to the worker for at least nine months before the worker's death. Furthermore, benefits to the surviving spouse are generally paid only if that person is not currently married, unless he or she did not remarry until after age 60.

A surviving spouse who is not yet 60 years old may be entitled to a mother's or father's benefit if he or she is caring for a child of the deceased worker who is either under age 16 or disabled (42 U.S.C. §402[g]). The benefit amount is equal to 75 percent of the deceased worker's benefit. A father or mother's benefit terminates if he or she remarries, when the surviving spouse becomes entitled to survivor benefits at age 60, or when the surviving spouse is eligible for Social Security retiree benefits.

Finally, there is a one-time payment of $255 to a surviving spouse. If the worker dies without a surviving spouse, the payment goes to any dependent children (42 U.S.C. §402[i]).

Children's Benefits

Children of a retiree can receive benefits if they are under 18 years of age, under 19 years of age and still attending elementary or high school, or over 18 years of age and disabled if the disability began before age 22 (42 U.S.C. §402[d]). A child includes natural children, adopted children, stepchildren, children born out of wedlock, and grandchildren. The legal definition of child can be expanded by claims of dependency. If the alleged parent claimed the child as a dependent on an income tax return, the child is entitled to child's benefits. To receive benefits, children must be unmarried and dependent upon the retiree for support.

A child's benefit is generally one-half of the retired worker's monthly benefit, but there is a family limit that caps the amount that Social Security will pay on any one worker's account. The family maximum does not affect the retired worker's own benefit, only the derivative benefits for spouse and children. Thus, the more children a retiree has, the smaller the benefit each child and his or her spouse will receive.

On the death of the retired worker, the benefits for any child who still qualifies rise to 75 percent of the retiree's benefit until the child outgrows age-based eligibility. Disabled children remain eligible so long as their disability continues.

Parental Benefits

Parents age 62 or older of a deceased worker are eligible for benefits based on the worker's earnings record if the parent receives at least one-half of his or her support from the worker (42 U.S.C. §402[h]). A "parent" includes natural parents and adoptive parents or stepparents who became such before the child reached age 16. Support means food, shelter, routine medical care, and other necessities.

Effect of Earnings after Retirement

Since 2000, a worker who reaches full retirement age can continue to work and receive the full amount of his or her retirement benefits. If you elect to take benefits before your full retirement age, an income test limits the amount of earnings you can receive before your Social Security benefits are reduced. This test includes only income from employment or self-employment and excludes income from other sources such as interest, dividends, or pensions.

Scope of Earnings

Income that triggers a reduction in your benefit includes any form of wages, salaries, bonuses, commissions, and net earnings from self-employment. Annuities, investment income, interest, pensions, and veterans or other government or military retirement benefits do not reduce Social Security benefits.

Applicable Thresholds

Once you reach full retirement age, your earnings have no effect on retirement benefits. Workers who claim benefits before reaching full retirement age have their benefits reduced $1 for every $2 earned above an earnings threshold ($14,160 in 2010) (42 U.S.C. §403[b]). This exempt earnings amount is adjusted annually for inflation. For example, Doris claims benefits at age 62. She works part time and earns $20,480, or $6,320 above the 2010 earnings limit. Her Social Security benefits will be reduced by $3,160.

In the year a worker reaches full retirement age, $1 in benefits will be deducted for each $3 earned above a higher earnings threshold ($37,680 in 2010). This exempt earnings threshold is also adjusted annually for inflation. Only earnings before the month when the worker reaches full retirement age are counted.

Effect on Derivative Benefits

The Social Security retirement earnings test is applied on an individual basis; a spouse's earnings are not considered in applying the earnings test to the retiree. However, if the benefits to the retiree are reduced due to excess earnings, any derivative benefits paid to a spouse or to any children will be reduced as well. The exception is for benefits to a divorced spouse, whose benefits are not affected by the reduction.

Taxation of Benefits

For most recipients, Social Security benefits are not taxed. However, approximately 25 percent of recipients are subject to a two-tiered federal income tax on benefits, based on the recipient's overall income (see 26 U.S.C. §86). This tax is triggered by income from any source, unlike the retirement earnings test, which considers only earned income. Individuals who do not have any earned income may still owe federal income tax on their Social Security benefits if their income from other sources is more than a certain amount. Income is calculated as the sum of

- adjusted gross income,
- tax-free interest income, and
- one-half of the recipient's Social Security benefits.

The tax on Social Security benefits is broken into two tiers. To be subject to the first tier of the tax, you must have income greater than $25,000 if single and $32,000 if married and filing a joint return. The amount in excess of the threshold is taxable, but under the first tier, no more than one-half of the recipient's Social Security benefits are taxed. To be subject to the second tier of the tax, a recipient must have income greater than $34,000 if single and $44,000 if married and filing a joint return. Eighty-five percent of the amount exceeding the threshold is added to the result from the first tier. This total amount is then taxable. At a maximum, no more than 85 percent of a recipient's Social Security benefits will be subject to taxation.

Disability Benefits

Disability benefits are payable to disabled workers as young as 21 years old. To qualify as disabled, the individual must be unable to perform any substantial gainful activity by reason of a medically established physical or mental impairment (42 U.S.C. §423[d]). The disability is determined by medical examinations, as well as vocational tests that assess whether a worker can be retrained for another type of employment. A disabled person can receive benefits up to full retirement age when the individual then begins receiving old-age benefits.

A disabled worker who receives workers compensation benefits may have his or her Social Security disability benefits reduced (42 U.S.C. §424a). This is known as the 80 percent rule because combined benefits cannot exceed 80 percent of the highest average monthly earnings in the five years preceding the onset of disability. If the combined benefits exceed 80 percent of the highest average monthly earnings, the Social Security benefits will be reduced so that total benefits will meet the 80 percent rule.

Application and Appeals Procedures

You can complete a Social Security benefit application online or at any of the SSA's local field offices. In general, you must provide proof of eligibility, such as proof of age, for the specific benefit sought. If your application is denied, SSA has a four-step process for contesting the determination (20 C.F.R. pt. 404, subpt. J). The field office handles the first step, in which it reconsiders initial determinations. The reconsideration is done by an employee of SSA who was not previously involved with the application. You may submit new evidence at this stage. The second step is a hearing before an administrative law judge within the SSA. The third step is a review of the administrative law judge's decision by the Appeals Council of the SSA. The Appeals Council can deny hearing on a case, remand the case back to the administrative law judge for further review, or hear the case and render a decision itself. Finally, you can seek judicial review in a federal district court.

Throughout the appeals process, you may have someone represent your interests. This person can be an attorney, but need not be. Other advocates, such as a union official, can represent a claimant.

Supplemental Security Income

If you are age 65 or older, blind, or disabled, and have very limited income and resources, you may be eligible for a federal cash assistance program known as Supplemental Security Income (SSI) (42 U.S.C. §1381a). Eligibility for SSI is very important because in most states it automatically qualifies you for Medicaid, the federal/state program of subsidized medical care (see Chapter 6 for a discussion of Medicaid eligibility), as well as for food stamps. Although SSI is funded and operated through the Social Security Administration, SSI eligibility differs from Social Security because it is based on financial need rather than your work record or the work record of your spouse. The following describes SSI benefits and eligibility requirements.

Benefits

SSI pays monthly cash benefits to qualified individuals and couples. The maximum benefit for an individual in 2010 was $674 per month, and the maximum benefit for a couple was $1,011 per month. Benefit amounts are adjusted annually for inflation. If you live in a nursing home or another institution with more than sixteen residents, your SSI benefit will be limited to a $30 per month personal needs allowance. Couples living in institutions can receive up to $60 per month.

If you live in someone else's household (for example, you live with an adult child), the benefit is reduced by one-third (20 C.F.R. §416.1131). This reduction is based on the presumption that you are receiving free food and shelter. The actual value of the items received is irrelevant. However, additional in-kind support will not cause a further reduction in benefits.

The one-third reduction will not apply if you pay your pro rata share of the cost of the room and food (20 C.F.R. §416.1133). The pro rata share is determined by dividing the average monthly household expenses, such as food, rent, property taxes, and utilities, by the number of persons in the household, regardless of age. For individuals who cannot pay their share of the expenses until they receive benefits, no reduction will be made if the person in charge of the household is only loaning the value of food and shelter with the expectation of repayment.

Another exception to the one-third reduction rule applies when the SSI recipient is a tenant in the house rather than merely living in someone else's household (20 C.F.R. §416.1132). This arrangement is viewed for SSI purposes as two separate households. Factors that establish separate household status include that the SSI recipient is not

- participating in household expenditure decisions,
- pooling money with others to meet expenses, and
- responsible for specific household bills.

All but five states supplement SSI benefits by providing additional monthly benefits.[3] Each state has its own criteria for determining who qualifies for such benefits and how much the state will pay. A number of states have the Social Security Administration administer payment of their state supplement.[4] If you live in one of these states, your state supplement will be included as a part of the SSI payment. No separate application for the state supplement is necessary.

In states that administer their own supplemental payment, you must apply for the supplement with the appropriate state agency. Some states pay supplements that depend on where the recipient is housed. Usually the objective of the state supplement is to help the recipient afford room and board in a setting such as a board and care home.

If you have an immediate need for either income or health care coverage, SSA may give emergency advance payments of SSI benefits. A onetime emergency advance payment may be made to address a financial emergency, which is defined as an immediate threat to health or safety, such as the inability to obtain food, clothing, shelter, or medical care. The amount of the emergency advance payment cannot exceed the federal benefit rate plus any available state supplement. Emergency advance payment amounts are recovered by SSA through proportionate reductions in SSI benefits over a period up to six months.

Eligibility for SSI Benefits

To be eligible for SSI, you must be a resident citizen of the United States or a qualified alien.[5] Illegal aliens are not eligible for SSI. If an SSI beneficiary is out of the country for more than thirty days, benefits are suspended until the beneficiary returns to the country (42 U.S.C. §1382[f]).

To receive SSI, you must file an application at a Social Security office or other authorized federal or state office (20 C.F.R. §416.305). Applicants are required to provide detailed information, including proof of income and resources, written authorization for the SSA to investigate their bank accounts, and proof of their living arrangements such as receipts and utility bills.

Applicants must also prove that they meet the SSI eligibility requirements as to age, blindness, or disability. To qualify based on age, you must prove that you are at least 65 years of age, verified by a public record such as a birth certificate, a religious birth record documented before age 5, or Immigration and Naturalization Service documents. If you are blind or disabled, you must submit to medical and vocational evaluations to substantiate those conditions. Applicants who knowingly provide false information or omit material information may have benefits suspended up to sixth months for the first offense, twelve months for the second offense, and twenty-four months for subsequent offenses.

Income Eligibility Requirements

Because SSI eligibility is based on financial need, there are strict income and asset rules that determine who is eligible (20 C.F.R. pt. 416, subpt. B). To receive benefits, your monthly income and assets must be below amounts set by the federal government. These amounts are adjusted annually for inflation.

Income eligibility is determined on a monthly basis. In 2010, to qualify for SSI an individual must have less than $674 in "countable income" per month, and a couple must have less than $1,011 (20 C.F.R. pt. 416, subpt. K).

Countable Income. Countable income is anything a person receives in cash or in-kind support that can be used to meet the need for food or shelter. It includes earned income, such as wages, and unearned income, such as pensions, Social Security, dividends, and interest (42 U.S.C. §1382a). Countable income even includes gifts. In-kind income may be earned, such as rent-free housing provided by an employer, or unearned, such as a gift of food. Whatever the form, all in-kind income that meets the need for food and shelter is countable income in determining eligibility for SSI. In-kind support that is not food or shelter, however, is not income and so does not count for determining SSI eligibility. For example, free medical or dental care is not considered income for SSI purposes, nor are gifts of a television or clothing.

SSI eligibility is determined monthly based on the countable income received two months previously. For example, SSI eligibility for March is determined by January's countable income. For initial eligibility, however, the countable income for the month in which SSI benefits are requested is used to determine SSI eligibility for that month and the next two months.

Not all income is countable income. The following are examples of some of the income that is not countable:

- value of food stamps
- home energy assistance
- state assistance
- disaster assistance
- loans that you have to repay
- income tax refunds
- food or shelter provided by nonprofit agencies

There are also exclusions from earned and unearned income used to arrive at the countable income figure for SSI eligibility. The monthly exclusion from unearned income is $20 and the monthly exclusion from earned income is $65. First, the $20 exclusion is subtracted from an applicant's unearned income, which is income other than wages, salary, or other employment compensation. For example, if you receive $70 per month in pension income, only $50 a month would be countable unearned income.

If you have less than $20 a month in unearned income, the $20 is subtracted from whatever unearned income you have, and the remainder is subtracted from your earned income. For example, if you have $15 a month in dividends and $125 a month in wages, the $20 is first subtracted from the unearned income of $15 ($15 − $20 = −$5), which leaves $5 to be deducted from the $125 of wages ($125 − $5 = $120). Then the $65 exclusion from earned income is subtracted from the $120 figure ($120 − $65 = $55), leaving $55 in earned income.

Once you have determined your earned income by this formula, one-half of whatever is left in earned income is then excluded. After the exclusions are taken out, the remaining earned income and unearned income figures are added together. If the sum is less than the maximum amount of the applicable monthly SSI benefit ($674 for individuals and $1,011 for couples in 2010), the individual or couple qualifies for SSI.

Consider the following example. Abby is single, age 67, and has no resources. She receives $200 a month from Social Security and has a part-time job that pays her $475 a month. The following calculations will be used to determine Abby's countable income:

Unearned income:	$200
Exclusion:	−20
	$180
Total countable unearned income = $180	
Earned income:	$475
Exclusion:	−65
	$410
	$410
Less one-half of earned income:	−205
	$205
Total countable earned income = $205	
Total countable income:	
Unearned	$180
Earned	+$205
	$385

Because the maximum monthly benefit in 2010 was $674, each $1 of countable income reduces Abby's SSI benefit by $1, yielding a monthly SSI benefit of $289 ($674 − $385 = $289) (20 C.F.R. §416.410).

Couples. The basic calculation of countable income for couples is the same but may be complicated by changing circumstances. For example, if an eligible individual becomes a couple with an ineligible spouse, the ineligible spouse's income is deemed to be available to the eligible spouse and is included in determining countable income. If both individuals are eligible and they separate, each will be paid at the individual rate (20 C.F.R. §416.432). If only one is eligible before separation, the income of the ineligible spouse will not be considered when determining benefits for the eligible spouse after separation. Couples need not be legally married under state law, but are considered married for SSI purposes if they live together and hold themselves out to the community as being married (42 U.S.C. §1382c[d][2]).

Resource Eligibility Requirements

Resources are cash, or liquid assets, and any real or personal property that an applicant could convert to cash for food and shelter. Individual applicants are ineligible for SSI if they have more than $2,000 in countable resources (20 C.F.R. §416.1205). Couples are excluded if they have more than $3,000 in countable resources (*id.*). Unlike income, however, resources that exceed the limits can be converted into exempt resources or spent down in order to make the applicant eligible, subject to the resource transfer rules to be discussed later in this chapter (20 C.F.R. pt. 416, subpt. L).

Some assets are partially or totally excluded from the eligibility test (42 U.S.C. §1382b). They include the following:

- the value of your home and the land on which it is located
- proceeds from the sale of the home if used to purchase another home within three months
- household goods and personal effects (but not investment property such as gems or collectibles)
- medical equipment
- the value of one vehicle if used for your transportation or that of your household members
- real or personal property necessary for self-support up to a value of $6,000 or items for self-support, such as a vegetable garden
- the value of burial plots for you and your immediate family
- up to $1,500 specifically set aside for burial expenses
- life insurance with a death value up to $1,500 (life insurance with a death value greater than $1,500 is a countable resource in the amount of its cash surrender value)
- cash received to be used to replace lost, damaged, or stolen excluded property if it is so used within nine months of receipt

The receipt of a lump sum such as an inheritance or lawsuit settlement is considered income in the month received. Any portion retained into the next month is considered a countable resource. A condition for receiving SSI benefits is the agreement to pursue all available sources of food and shelter. Therefore, an individual cannot renounce an inheritance to acquire or maintain eligibility for SSI.

If the individual has resources that exceed the limit, he or she may still begin to receive SSI benefits immediately if the following conditions exist:

- Total excess liquid resources, such as cash, do not exceed one-fourth of the dollar amount of the basic federal benefit.
- The applicant agrees to dispose of the excess nonliquid resources within nine months if real property and within three months if personal property (the three-month period can be extended another three months for good cause) (20 C.F.R. §416.1245).

The individual will not be forced to sell a jointly owned house if its sale would cause an undue hardship because the other owner lives in the house or if attempts to sell the house have been unsuccessful. An undue hardship means that no other housing is readily available.

Resource Transfer Rules. An individual or couple who gives away countable resources may be ineligible for SSI. On application for SSI, you must account for any transfer that was for less than fair market value during the thirty-six months preceding the application (42 U.S.C. §1382b[c]). You will not be eligible for a period of time equal to the value of the transferred resources divided by the federal SSI payment rate and the state supplement, if any, up to a maximum of thirty-six months. The penalty period begins to run in the month of the transfer.

For example, Mel, age 68, gave $3,100 to his daughter on May 1, 2009. The period for which he is ineligible for SSI is five months ($3,100 ÷ $674 = 4.6 months [the period is rounded to the nearest whole number]). If a married applicant makes a transfer that results in a period of ineligibility, and then the spouse becomes eligible for benefits, the penalty is divided between the applicant and the spouse.

SSA presumes that transfer or disposal of assets for less than fair market value was made to establish initial or continued eligibility for SSI benefits. An individual can challenge that presumption by presenting evidence that the transfer was for a purpose other than creating eligibility. Transfers that were not made with the intent of qualifying for benefits can be reversed and the penalty avoided if the resources are returned. Where a transfer penalty would impose a hardship, the SSA can waive the penalty.

Certain transfers are exempt from the transfer penalties. Transfers to or for the sole benefit of the spouse do not create a period of ineligibility. Other exempt transfers include the transfer of a home to a spouse, a child under age 21, a child who is blind or disabled, a sibling with an interest in the house who has resided there for more than one year prior to the applicant entering an institution, or a child who resided in the home for a period of at least two years immediately prior to the applicant entering an institution and who provided care to the applicant that delayed the applicant's entry into an institution (42 U.S.C. §1382b[c][1][C][i]).

Notes

1. For more information on calculating quarters of coverage, see 20 C.F.R. §404.140-146.

2. Social Security Amendments of 1983, Pub. L. No. 98-21, 97 Stat. 65 (1983) (codified as amended in scattered sections of 42 U.S.C.).

3. Arkansas, Kansas, Mississippi, Tennessee, and West Virginia do not provide additional benefits.

4. These states are California, Delaware, District of Columbia, Hawaii, Iowa, Massachusetts, Michigan, Montana, Nevada, New Jersey, New York, Pennsylvania, Rhode Island, Utah, and Vermont.

5. There are seven categories of noncitizens who are qualified aliens as determined by the Department of Homeland Security. Qualified aliens must meet additional requirements for SSI eligibility beyond being aged, blind, or disabled and having limited income and resources (8 U.S.C. §1612[a]).

For More Information

Social Security Administration (800-772-1213)
(http://www.ssa.gov)

Find information about retirement, disability, and SSI benefits. The site provides guidance concerning online applications as well as the location of local Social Security offices. There are also tools to help you estimate benefits and make decisions about when to begin receiving retirement benefits.

4
Employer-Provided Retirement Benefits and IRAs

Did You Know?

- You could owe a 10 percent penalty tax if you withdraw retirement benefits before age 59½.
- You can receive early distributions from your individual retirement account (IRA) without penalty if the money is for the higher education expenses of yourself, your spouse, your child, or your grandchild.
- You could owe a penalty if you *fail* to begin taking benefits from your retirement plan and IRAs after you reach age 70½.
- Distributions from most retirement plans are taxable to the recipient, even when the recipient is the spouse or beneficiary of a retiree who dies.
- If you leave your job after you are vested in the retirement plan, you may be able to roll over your benefits into an individual IRA without tax consequences.

Most Americans look forward to a time when they can retire. After a lifetime of work, they hope to enjoy their later years without the burden of a daily job. Of course, retirement means the loss of a steady paycheck, and so seniors must have another source of income. Social Security benefits are a start, and many seniors will save for their retirement. Most seniors expect to receive retirement benefits from their former employer. In reality, only about one-half of retirees enjoy retirement benefits other than Social Security benefits.

This chapter discusses the laws that govern retiree pensions and retirement benefits such as 401(k) plans. All private employer–sponsored retirement benefit plans are exclusively governed by federal law, the Employee Retirement Insurance Security Act enacted in 1974, commonly referred to as ERISA (29 U.S.C. §§1001 *et seq.*). Federal law preempts any state law in this area, meaning that states cannot attempt to regulate employee pension, retirement, or welfare benefit plans in a way that is inconsistent with federal law. ERISA, however, does not govern pension plans sponsored by public entities such as states and cities.

ERISA defines two basic types of employee benefit plans: (1) "employee pension benefit plans" or "pension plans" and (2) "employee welfare benefit plans" or "welfare plans" (29 U.S.C. §1002[1], [2], [3]). Employer-offered benefit plans, both pension and welfare, are also regulated under the Internal Revenue Code (IRC), which grants very favorable tax treatment to those plans that meet a number of detailed requirements. Plans that receive favorable tax treatment are called "qualified" plans because they meet the qualifications required by the IRC.

Pension plans are created by employers to provide employees with retirement income after the employee reaches a certain age and ends employment with the employer. In contrast, welfare plans provide employees, and sometimes retirees, with a variety of benefits, the most important of which are health, disability, and life insurance. Health care insurance is by far the most important and valuable benefit offered by employer-provided welfare plans.

Pension and Retirement Plans

Employee pension benefit plans are further defined by ERISA as either "defined benefit plans" or "defined contribution plans"(29 U.S.C. §1002[34], [35]). For the purposes of this book, the term "pension plan" is used interchangeably with the term "defined benefit plan" to refer to plans that provide lifetime benefits, usually a fixed monthly payment for life. The term "retirement plan" is used interchangeably with "defined contribution plan" to refer to plans that provide a lump-sum dollar amount to the employee upon retirement. Employers can offer both pension and retirement plans. The following examples illustrate the difference.

Jill worked for Alpha Inc., which provides its retired employees with a *pension plan* equal to 60 percent of their last year's earnings. Jill earned $50,000 her last year before she retired, and so she will be paid $30,000 a year for life (60% x $50,000 = $30,000). In contrast, Jason worked for Beta Inc., a company with a *retirement plan* to which it contributes an amount equal to 5 percent of the employee's wages. The funds in this account are payable to that employee upon retirement. Jason has worked for Beta Inc. for thirty years, during which time each pay period Beta contributed 5 percent of his wages to his retirement account. Upon Jason's retirement at age 65, he is entitled to his retirement account worth $472,300.

This chapter discusses the important differences between pension and retirement plans and provides information on related topics such as normal retirement age (NRA), vesting requirements, 401(k) plans, and the role of IRAs.

Defined Benefit or Pension Plans

Defined benefit plans are pension plans that promise participating employees a specified monthly pension benefit at retirement. Most defined benefit plans do not promise a particular dollar amount; rather, they promise a benefit determined by a formula. This formula is based on the employee's number of years of employment and his or her rate of pay.

Consider the following example. John works for Chi Company, which offers a plan that will pay a pension for life. The formula used by Chi to determine the benefit amount for its retirees is the employee's average pay for the last three years of employment multiplied by a percentage based on the number of years of employment. Chi Company uses a factor of 1.5 to determine this percentage. At age 65 John retires. He has worked for Chi Company for thirty years, and his average pay for the last three years of employment was $60,000. His pension is computed as follows: 30 years x 1.5 = 45%; 45% x $60,000 = $27,000. After his retirement at age 65, John will receive a yearly pension of $27,000 for life.

Some employees, such as construction workers, work for a variety of firms over their careers. In industries where employees work for various employers, the employers may contribute to a common defined benefit plan known as a "multiemployer" pension plan (29 U.S.C. §1002[37][A]). Typically this is available when the employees are members of a union that bargains for a pension plan on behalf of its members. A multiemployer plan operates like any defined benefit plan. Over the working life of the employee, the various employers contribute to a single defined benefit pension plan. The plan pays benefits based upon a formula that treats the employees as if they had worked for a single employer during their careers.

Regardless of how a defined benefit pension is calculated, payments are made for the life of the employee and, if the employee is married, until both the employee and the spouse have died (unless the spouse has waived his or her rights under the pension) (29 U.S.C. §1055). For married retirees, the amount of the monthly payment is often reduced because the benefit will likely be paid for more years. For example, Hank and Tom have both been employed by Sigma Inc. for thirty years and have identical pay histories. They share the same birthday and retire on the same date. Hank is single. According to the formula used to determine pensions, he is entitled to $25,000 a year for life. If Tom were single, he, too, would receive $25,000 a year for life. Tom, however, is married to Tina and so will receive a joint life annuity, meaning that the annuity will be paid until the last of the two dies. As a result, Tom's pension is reduced to $18,000 a year because, taken together, Tom and Tina have a longer life expectancy than does Hank. Although employers are not required to reduce the benefit paid to a husband and wife, they typically do.

In a defined benefit plan, the employer each year contributes the amount that is estimated as necessary to ensure enough plan assets to pay the benefits promised to employees. The employer contributions are held in a trust fund and invested, usually in stocks and bonds. The investment earnings are added to the fund and help pay for the promised pensions.

Actuaries, using estimates of how many years employees can be expected to work, their estimated average compensation when they retire, and the expected rate of investment return on the plan assets determine how much the employer must contribute each year. The rate of return on the investments is a critical component in determining how much the employer must contribute to the pension fund. Because the fund invests its assets and earns income, the employer does not have to contribute every dollar that will eventually be paid in benefits.

The greater the earnings are by a defined benefit plan fund, the fewer are the dollars the employer will need to contribute to the fund. In some years, the employer will not need to pay any money to the fund because the earnings on the fund will have exceeded what the actuary estimated is needed. In other years, the investments of the fund will not have produced as much income as expected. This means that the employer will have to contribute more to make up for the shortfall. Because employer contributions vary based upon the fund's investment earnings, defined benefit plans place the risk of how well the plan investments perform upon the employer. Regardless of how well the plan investments perform, the employee benefits do not vary. The employer contributions to the plan cannot be returned to the employer unless the plan is terminated and there is more money in the plan than is needed to pay off all the promised employee pensions (29 U.S.C. §1344).

A defined benefit plan can be "integrated" with Social Security, meaning that benefits paid by the plan to an employee are reduced to reflect in part the benefits that the employee receives from Social Security (I.R.C. §401[a][5][D]). Integration, which lowers the cost of plans for the employer, is complicated and subject to complex statutory and regulatory requirements, but the bottom line is that integrated plans pay fewer benefits than do nonintegrated plans.

Another form of defined benefit pension plan that is growing in popularity with employers is the "cash balance plan." In a cash balance plan, the employer makes an annual contribution to a pension account for the employee based upon a formula, typically a percentage of the employee's compensation. The employer also announces an investment rate of return. This rate is not the actual investment return on the plan fund, but rather the rate that will determine the annual amount credited to the fund. For example, the plan may announce that it will credit employees' accounts with an annual compounded rate of return of 6 percent. Even though each account will be credited with the announced rate of return, in reality the rate of investment return on the collective fund could be higher or lower. If the actual rate of return is higher than the announced rate of return, the excess investment income does not benefit the employees but rather reduces the employer's required annual contribution. If the actual return is lower, the employer must make up the difference.

Employers that offer a cash balance pension plan try to select an announced rate of return that they are confident the plan investments can earn. For example, they might select the interest rate on U.S. Treasury bonds. Upon retirement, the employee is paid a lump sum equal to the contributions made by the employer plus the announced rate of return.

Defined Contribution or Retirement Plans

Retirement plans are quite different from pension plans. Called defined contribution plans, they do not promise any set amount of benefits. Rather, the employer promises to place a set amount aside in an account for the benefit of the employee. Each year of employment that the plan is in effect, the employer adds an additional amount to the employee's retirement account. The account is invested in stocks, bonds, and other investments, and the earnings are added to the account of the employee. On the date the employee retires (leaves the employment of the employer) and has reached the designated retirement age, the employee is given access to his or her retirement account.

Payment options under retirement plans vary from employer to employer. Depending on the plan rules, the employee will either be able to withdraw all the money in the retirement account or use that money to purchase a lifetime annuity. For example, Betty has worked for Delta Inc. for the last thirty years. Each year, pursuant to the company's retirement plan, Delta placed an amount equal to 3 percent of Betty's annual wages into her retirement account. It invested the account, and the earnings from that investment were added to the account. When Betty left the company at age 62 (the earliest year in which she could access her account), her account had a total value of $210,000. Under the terms of the plan, Betty could either withdraw the entire $210,000 or she could purchase a lifetime annuity that would pay her $15,000 a year for life.

Under a traditional defined contribution plan, the employer names a plan administrator or trustee who has the responsibility for managing the plan, which includes investing the employee accounts and distributing the benefits to the retired employees. The defined contribution plan combines all the funds for the employees into a single investment account. The employees have no control as to how the fund is invested; that is the duty of the plan administrator. Employer contributions to the plan cannot be returned to the employer.

A defined contribution plan places the risk of success of the plan's investment upon the employees. The employer only promises to contribute a set amount and makes no promises as to how rapidly the amount will grow. The amount the employee will eventually receive depends heavily on how well the investments of the defined contribution plan perform. The greater the earnings are, the greater is the employee's retirement benefit. For example, Kathy works for Delta Inc. and Kent works for Epsilon Inc. Both are paid the same wage, and both companies contribute an amount equal to 5 percent of their wages to a defined contribution plan. Kathy's account, managed by the Delta fund over her twenty-five-year work history, has an average investment return of 7 percent. During Kent's twenty-five-year work history, the Epsilon plan has an average rate of return of only 5 percent. As a result, when Kathy and Kent retire at the same time, Kathy's lump-sum distribution is $500,000, whereas Kent's is only $400,000.

Employee stock ownership plans (ESOPs) are a particular type of defined contribution plan. An ESOP creates individual accounts for each participant that are funded primarily with the employer's stock, and the benefits are generally paid in the form of employer stock. For example, Lisa works for Alpha Company, which operates an ESOP. The ESOP fund consists of 85 percent Alpha Company stock and 15 percent U.S. Treasury bonds. When Lisa retires, she will receive a distribution that will consist almost exclusively of Alpha Company stock, which she can then sell or continue to hold.

Because ERISA is supposed to promote fairness and greater employee participation in pension and retirement plans, it limits an employer's ability to exclude certain employees from pension and retirement plans and restricts the employer's authority to discriminate against lower-paid employees with respect to benefits. For example, a company cannot operate a qualified pension or retirement plan—a plan that enjoys the federal income tax advantages of a qualified plan—if the plan covers only the higher-paid management employees. The act contains complex nondiscrimination rules that generally require a plan to benefit at least 70 percent of non–highly compensated employees so that the plan does not disproportionately benefit highly compensated employees such as the company officers (I.R.C. §401[a][4]).

Normal Retirement Age

If you participate in an employer-sponsored pension or retirement plan, you cannot receive retirement benefits from it until you have reached the normal retirement age stated in the plan. An NRA cannot be later than either age 65 or ten years after you start work. For example, Alpha Inc. has an NRA of age 65, but Tom begins to work for Alpha at age 58. Alpha can use age 68 (ten years after Tom's start date) as Tom's NRA. When you reach the NRA, you may, but are not required to, retire and collect your retirement benefits.

To retire means only that you quit your job with your employer. It does not mean that you have to stop working altogether. You can quit, collect retirement benefits, and find a new job. For example, Carol works for Beta Inc., which has a defined benefit pension plan with an NRA of age 62. Carol turns age 62 and retires from Beta Inc. and begins to collect her defined benefit pension. She then goes to work for Kappa Company. Her employment with Kappa Company will not affect her right to collect her monthly pension from Beta Inc.

If you quit before you reach the NRA, you cannot collect any benefits until you reach the NRA. For example, Dale also works for Beta Inc. After thirty years of working for Beta Inc., Dale quits at age 60 and does not take another job. He must wait until he turns age 62 to begin to collect his pension from Beta Inc. The same is true for Emily, who quits at age 42 after working for Beta Inc. for ten years. She has earned a pension by virtue of her ten years of employment, but she must wait twenty years, until she turns 62, to collect it.

If you continue to work past the NRA, you will continue to earn additional pension benefits, subject to any plan limits. The plan, for example, may cap the number of years of employment used to determine the size of your pension. For example, Ed, age 68, has worked thirty-seven years for Kappa Company, which has a pension plan with an NRA of age 65 and a thirty-five-year limit on the number of countable years used to calculate the defined benefit pension. No matter how many years above thirty-five Ed actually works at Kappa, his pension will be calculated as if he had worked there for only thirty-five years.

Defined benefit plans sometimes have an NRA of 65 and an alternative trigger for benefits based on a combination of the employee's age and years of employment. For example, the plan might permit employees to qualify for their pension whenever the combination of their age and number of years of employment totals a designated number, such as ninety. Fred is age 60 and has worked for the employer for thirty years. He can retire and begin his pension payments because the total of his age plus the number of years worked adds up to ninety.

Plans may offer survivor's benefits to family members of employees who die before they have retired or reached the NRA. Some plans pay a lump-sum death benefit to surviving spouses or heirs of a deceased employee. Plans may also pay a disability pension to a disabled employee until he or she reaches the normal retirement age and is eligible for the retirement pension.

Vesting

Under ERISA, employees must become "vested" to receive retirement benefits. Vesting means that an employee's retirement benefits cannot be lost or forfeited once he or she has participated in the plan for a prescribed number of years—typically five years or on a graduated basis over seven years (29

U.S.C. §1053). After an employee is vested, termination of employment will not mean the loss of the pension. For example, Garth worked for Beta Inc. from 1990 to 2000 and quit before he reached the plan NRA of 62. When Garth turns age 62, he will be eligible for whatever retirement benefits he earned while employed with Beta.

Note that Garth could have vested pension benefit plans from more than one employer. Suppose that after he left Beta Inc. he went to work for Rho Company for ten years and earned a vested pension payable at the NRA of age 62. When Garth turns age 62, he can begin to collect pensions from both Beta Inc. and Rho Company.

Like defined benefit plans, defined contribution plans also provide for vesting after a minimum number of years of participation, usually five, but as long as seven. If you terminate employment after being vested, the value of your retirement account will continue to grow according to the success of the plan's investments until you withdraw the value of the account. You can withdraw money from a defined contribution account operated by a former employer at any age, but because of income tax advantages (discussed later in the chapter), you would be wise not to withdraw funds until you have reached at least age 59½.

In the past, defined benefit plans were the most commonly offered form of pension or retirement plan, but they have lost favor in recent years and now represent fewer than 20 percent of all plans. The greatest attraction of a defined benefit for employees is the knowledge that the longer they work for the employer, the larger will be their pensions. Employees also like that at any time they can calculate their future benefits. For example, if you expect to retire at age 62 under a defined benefit pension plan, at age 60 you could estimate pretty closely what your monthly benefit is likely to be by plugging numbers into the pension formula. Many employers with defined benefit plans provide their workers with annual estimates of individual employee projected pension benefits.

Employees who change employers frequently or who are not sure how long they will stay with their present employer are less attracted to defined benefit plans. Suppose, for example, that during your work career you work for three companies, Alpha, Beta, and Chi, each for ten years. You are vested in each company's defined benefit plan, and each uses the same formula to determine your retirement pension. The formula is (2% × the number of years employed) × (your average wage for the last two years of employment). In other words, based on ten years of employment, you will receive a 20 percent replacement (2% × 10 yrs.) of your average ending wage. Suppose that your average wage during the last two years of employment at Alpha was $40,000; at Beta, $50,000; and at Chi, $70,000. Your Alpha pension will be $8,000, your Beta pension will be $10,000, and your Chi pension will be $14,000, for a total of $32,000.

Now assume that you had spent all thirty years of your career with the same employer, Alpha, and had averaged $70,000 a year for the last two years of employment. You would have been credited with thirty years of employment multiplied by 2 percent for a multiplier of 60 percent (instead of 20 percent). At 60 percent of your $70,000 average wage, your pension would be $42,000 a year, or $10,000 more than it was when you worked for three employers.

The defined benefit plan pension is clearly most beneficial to employees who have only one or two employers in their lifetime of work. That employment pattern, however, is much less common today than in the past. Today's employees frequently change jobs, with the result that fewer employees are able to earn a substantial defined benefit pension. Consider the different outcome in our example if Alpha, Beta, and Chi all had defined contribution, rather than defined benefit, plans. Assuming that each had contributed the same percentage of your wages to a defined contribution plan, you would have the same amount in your account (provided that each had the same investment return) as if you had worked for just one of them for the entire thirty years.

Employers have also come to prefer defined contribution plans, both because they are less costly to administer and because today's employer does not expect that most employees will stay with one employer for the majority of their careers. The decline of unions, which often insisted on defined benefit plans, has also contributed to the decline of such plans. The main reason, however, that employers have turned to defined contribution plans is that such plans shift the risk of the plan investments to the employee. If a defined benefit plan has poor investment returns, the employer will have to make additional contributions to the plan in order to meet its pension obligations. In contrast, if a defined contribution plan has poor investment returns, only the employees suffer.

401(k) Plans

The fastest growing form of retirement plan is the 401(k) plan, which is a form of defined contribution plan named after the Internal Revenue Code section that authorizes it. More than one-half of all retirement plans and an overwhelming majority of new plans are 401(k) plans. The plans are very popular because the employee, rather than the employer, directs how the employee's retirement account is invested.

A 401(k) plan is a "cash or deferred arrangement" (CODA) that gives employees the choice whether to receive all of their wages now as cash wages or to have a portion of their wages contributed to a retirement plan account. If the employee elects to receive all of his or her wages now, the amount received is taxable income. However, if the employee elects to have part of his or her wages contributed to a retirement account, the retirement account contribution is not currently taxed. This tax advantage is designed to encourage employees to contribute to their retirement accounts. The employer can either make the contribution to the retirement account automatic, though reversible by the employee, or the default can be that the employees receive the cash unless they authorize it to be paid to the retirement 401(k) account (I.R.C. §401[k][2][A]). Contribution rates to 401(k) accounts are much higher if employees are automatically enrolled and contributions made on their behalf unless they choose not to contribute.

The amount that an employee can contribute each year to a 401(k) account is limited, with the limit adjusted annually for inflation. In 2010 the amount was $16,500. 401(k) plans are also subject to limitations on contributions by what the statute refers to as "highly compensated employees," typically the company executives, so that the rate of participation by these employees is not excessive compared to the rates of participation by the non–highly compensated employees (I.R.C. §401[k][3]). Employee contributions to 401(k) plans are immediately vested (I.R.C. §401[a][3]). That is, the employee will not lose his or her contributions even if the employee does not remain with the company long enough to become vested in matching amounts contributed by the employer.

Typically, a 401(k) plan permits employees to contribute up to some percentage of their wages. For example, the plan might permit a 3 percent contribution (up to the annual limit). In addition, many employers offer matching contributions. For example, suppose the plan provides for a 50 percent employer match of the employee's contribution. If you contribute 3 percent of your wages to your 401(k), a 50 percent employer match means that your employer will contribute another 1.5 percent. Neither the amounts contributed by the employer nor the amounts contributed by you are taxed until you later take distributions from your account.

When you take money out of your 401(k) account, it will be taxable income. If you take it out too soon, it will be taxed and also subject to an additional 10 percent penalty tax (I.R.C. §72[t]). Withdrawals of money are not subject to the penalty if the withdrawal does not occur until after the earliest of

- termination of employment from the employer that sponsors the plan after age 55 in conjunction with an early retirement plan,
- reaching of age 59½,
- death or disability,
- the occurrence of an immediate and pressing financial hardship, or
- reaching of the plan's NRA, which cannot be later than age 65 (29 U.S.C. §1002[24]).

Most withdrawals occur after the employee has reached age 59½ and is no longer working for the employer. Once you have reached the NRA, you can begin to take money out of the plan without the penalty tax even if you are still working for the employer who sponsored the plan. Your employer may have an early retirement plan that would permit you to withdraw funds from your 401(k) plan without the 10 percent penalty as early as age 55.

If you terminate employment with the plan sponsor before age 59½ or the normal retirement age, and you do not want to be taxed on a distribution from the 401(k), you can do either of the following:

- Leave the 401(k) account with that employer's 401(k) plan, and begin withdrawing funds from it when you reach age 59½ or the normal retirement age of the plan (subject to federal income taxation on the distributions at that time).
- Roll over the 401(k) account to an IRA that you manage (although you cannot receive money from the IRA without penalty until you reach age 59½) (I.R.C. §402[c]).

If you have a 401(k) account, you can participate in decisions about how the funds are invested, but your employer is permitted to limit your investment choices. The plan as created by the employer must offer a choice of at least three different, diversified investment options, and the plan must permit participants to transfer their assets among the three options at least every three months (29 U.S.C. §1104[c]; 29 C.F.R. §2550.404c-1[b]). Very commonly, 401(k) plans permit employees to choose among investing in bank certificates of deposit, bonds, the stock of the employer, and one or more designated mutual funds. Some plans simply permit the employee to invest in a "family" of diversified funds offered by an investment firm. Whatever the permitted choices, your employer is not liable if the investments that you choose decline in value or fail to perform as you had hoped.

Unfortunately, many 401(k) participants are not very knowledgeable about how to invest. They tend to be too conservative in their investments, investing too much in bank certificates of deposit and bonds and not enough in stocks, and so they earn a relatively low rate of return. Commonly, the employee will fail to reallocate investments and just stay with the original investment choices.

Another potential problem with 401(k) plans is that employees are permitted to borrow funds from their accounts (29 U.S.C. §1108[b][1]). While the money is out on loan, it is not growing as an investment. In some cases, the employee will never pay back the loan, with the result that the loan becomes taxable income and may be subject to the additional 10 percent penalty tax. Thus, mediocre investment results, unpaid loans from 401(k) accounts, and a failure of some employees to fully participate in the plan are some of the reasons that many employees are going to retire with only modest retirement accounts and without the economic security they will need in their later years.

Another practice that can result in poor retirement plan performance is the employer contribution of company stock, rather than cash, to match employee contributions. Employees may also be encouraged to purchase employer stock with their 401(k) contributions. As a result, many employee retirement accounts are much too concentrated in the stock of the employer. Any long-term investment should be well diversified. Investing too much in your employer's stock carries a double risk. If your employer gets into financial difficulty, not only is your job at risk, but also the value of your 401(k) account will fall. It is simply common sense not to bet both your job and your retirement investment account on the same employer.

A factor that can add to the risk of investment in employer stock is the employer practice of setting time limits on when employees can sell employer stock. For example, some employers prohibit the sale of contributed stock for five or even ten years. In the severe stock market decline of the early 2000s, many employees were unable to sell a significant proportion of their 401(k) assets because of employer time limits on the selling of the employer-contributed company stock. As a result, employees were helpless to divest or sell off stock that was rapidly losing value, some even to the point of having to retain the stock while the employer went bankrupt. The result was devastating losses of 401(k) retirement funds for many employees. Nonetheless, ERISA generally does not prohibit employers from restricting participants in the sale of company stock.

Despite some of the potential problems with 401(k) plans, they have the great advantage of being portable. Because all of your contributions to your 401(k) are immediately vested, the account belongs to you no matter what happens. Even if you are fired or quit, you continue to own the account and direct the investments until you finally take distributions from it. If you stop working for the employer who sponsored your 401(k), you have the option to leave it alone, to transfer it to a new 401(k) account offered by your new employer, or to "roll over" your 401(k) investments into an IRA that you own and whose investments are directed by you (I.R.C. §408[d][3]). If you roll over the account within sixty days of termination of your employment, the transfer is not subject to federal income tax. The returns on the investments by the IRA continue to be free of income tax until finally distributed to you. Over your work career, you could roll over several 401(k) accounts to an IRA as you move from job to job.

Some employers permit employees to convert their 401(k) accounts to "Roth" accounts. Even though the amounts placed in a Roth 401(k) are taxed as income, all future distributions from the account are tax free, including all the investment income earned by the account. For taxation purposes, you can think of a Roth 401(k) as just the opposite of the traditional 401(k). In a traditional 401(k) the contributions are excluded from income taxation, but the distributions (including any earnings) are eventually taxed.

With a Roth account, the contributions are subject to income taxation, but the earnings and distributions are not.

Qualified Plans

Qualified plans are retirement plans that receive favorable federal income tax treatment because they meet the complex requirements of the Internal Revenue Code. This favorable tax treatment is meant to promote employer-provided pension and retirement plans. Nonqualified plans are those plans that do not meet these requirements and do not receive favorable tax treatment.

Qualified plans enjoy three significant income tax advantages:

1. The employer may deduct from its taxable income contributions made to the plan (I.R.C. §404[a][1],[2], [3]).
2. Though the employer takes a tax deduction for contributions, the employees do not report any income or pay any tax until distributions are actually paid to them (I.R.C. §402[a]).
3. Investment earnings on the retirement account funds are not taxed until paid out to the employee (I.R.C. §501[a]).

How Pension and Retirement Plans Operate

Employers are not required to create or operate pension or retirement plans, and about one-half of all employers do not. Moreover, the employer has the right to change or terminate the plan at any time. An employer that has decided to create a pension or retirement plan is a "plan sponsor" and decides whether the plan will be a defined benefit, cash balance, or defined contribution plan. The employer also decides which employees will be included in the plan. Absent a collective bargaining agreement with a union, employers are granted by federal law a fair amount of discretion as to whom to include in the plan. A qualified retirement plan may exclude employees under age 21 and may also require an employee to complete one year of employment before becoming eligible to join the plan (29 U.S.C. §1052). The plan can also exclude classes of employees. Often an employer will exclude union members because the union members may have collectively bargained for a separate pension plan. Some employers exclude a particular job classification. A law firm, for example, might exclude messengers from participating in its plan, which is otherwise open to all the other staff and all the attorneys.

If the plan is a defined benefit plan, the employer must determine the benefit formula. For a defined contribution plan, it must decide on the amount of the employer contribution or whether to adopt a 401(k) plan. The employer must also determine the kind of distributions the plan will pay, such as lump-sum distributions or annuities.

The employer, as plan sponsor, must name a plan administrator, who may be a single individual or several persons. The plan administrator will be responsible for managing the plan, including identifying who is eligible, overseeing the investments, paying the benefits, filing required governmental reports, and maintaining the plan records. The plan sponsor can name itself as the plan administrator, and many do. Others name banks or other institutions as the plan administrator. Some name corporate officers, such as the vice president for finance.

ERISA requires that retirement benefits become vested no later than seven years after the employee started employment. Employees must be allowed to join the retirement plan at least by the time they reach age 21 or have been employed for one year, whichever comes later. However, a pension plan may require three years of employment for eligibility if at the end of those three years the employee also immediately becomes 100 percent vested (29 U.S.C. §1052).

Spousal Benefits

ERISA requires that qualified plans offer joint and survivor annuities for married employees. A joint and survivor annuity pays a retirement benefit until both spouses have died, unless that right was specifically waived in writing by the employee and the spouse (29 U.S.C. §1055). To reject the survivor option, both the employee and the spouse must sign a written waiver that is witnessed by a plan representative or notary public. The employee has ninety days to change his or her mind and revoke the waiver of spousal rights.

Normally qualified plan benefits cannot be assigned for payment to creditors or other third parties. The only exception is that the benefits can be subject to a state qualified domestic relations order (QDRO) (29 U.S.C. §1056[d][3]). Under a QDRO, pension rights can be altered and reassigned. For example, the QDRO could provide that the divorced spouse of the plan participant, rather than the current spouse, will be treated as the surviving spouse for purposes of receiving the survivor's annuity after the death of the plan participant. Or the benefits under the plan might be made payable to the former spouse, rather than to the employee.

Payment of Benefits

When you qualify and apply for benefits under a pension or retirement plan, you will either receive a lump-sum amount or a lifetime annuity. If you are married, the plan must pay an annuity until both you and your spouse have died, unless your spouse waived the right to the annuity. Plans often purchase annuities for retired employees from an insurance company, which in turn pays the lifetime annuity to the retired employee.

In the case of a 401(k) plan, upon your retirement you have the right to withdraw the entire value of the account, but of course any amounts withdrawn are subject to federal income taxation. In many cases, it would be much wiser to roll the 401(k) funds over into an IRA and then take annual distributions from the IRA. Once you reach age 70½, the Internal Revenue Code requires that you take a minimum distribution from your retirement plan or IRA to ensure that tax-deferred funds do not go untaxed indefinitely.

If you have a defined benefit plan, the amount of the monthly payment under the annuity contract will depend on the formula adopted by the employer when it created the plan. If the actuarial value of an employee's benefits at the date of termination is worth $5,000 or less, the plan can pay the employee the actuarial value of the vested pension rather than an annuity (I.R.C. §417[e][1]).

If you participate in a defined contribution plan, upon retirement you will either receive a lump sum that represents the value of your account or the plan may permit the lump sum to be converted into a lifetime annuity, much as if it were a defined benefit plan. The lump sum will be used to purchase an annuity that will pay a monthly benefit in an amount that is determined by your life expectancy (without regard to sex) or, if you are married, by the combined life expectancy of you and your spouse and the value of your defined contribution account. The older you are and the greater the value of your defined contribution account is, the larger will be your monthly annuity benefit. Employees who participate in a defined contribution plan and who terminate employment before their retirement date eventually receive their vested retirement benefits when they reach the plan's normal retirement age.

Under the Internal Revenue Code, the employer may permit employees who have reached the age of 55 to take early retirement and receive their retirement benefits without imposition of the 10 percent penalty tax. Employers often use early retirement as a way to reduce the number of employees and thereby reduce their payroll because doing so encourages older, more highly paid employees to voluntarily leave. For example, Beta Inc.'s normal retirement age for its defined benefit plan is 62. Beta Inc. needs to reduce its workforce by 10 percent. To do so, it permits employees age 55 or older to take early retirement and begin to collect their pension. Even though the amount of the pension is less than if they continued to work until age 62, many prefer to retire. Others elect to take early retirement because they fear that if they do not, the company will fire many employees and they might be one of those fired. Employees who are involuntarily terminated would not be able to collect their pension until they reach the NRA of age 62.

Absent the exclusion for early retirement, if an employee receives benefits before age 59½, the benefits are subject to the federal income tax plus a penalty tax equal to 10 percent of the amount withdrawn. The penalty tax does not apply to benefits paid to

- a beneficiary or an estate of a deceased employee,
- a disabled employee, or
- an alternate payee pursuant to a QDRO, or to
- payments that are part of a series of substantially equal periodic payments made for the life of the employee, such as an annuity (I.R.C. §72[t][2]).

Nonqualified Employer-Provided Plans

Nonqualified employer-provided plans do not enjoy the federal income tax advantages of qualified plans. In essence, a nonqualified plan is merely a deferred income arrangement. Employees sometimes want deferred income because they anticipate that after they retire, they will be taxed at a lower rate. Employers may offer a nonqualified plan along with qualified plans when the employer wishes to provide additional deferred compensation to a limited number of employees, such as highly paid executives. Nonqualified plans permit an employer to supplement an employee's benefit package without violating the nondiscrimination rules of qualified plans or being bound by the funding limits imposed on qualified plans.

If the nonqualified plan is not funded and is merely a promise to pay benefits to the employee at a later date, the employees are not taxed until they actually receive the benefits. Of course, the employee takes the risk that the employer will not be able to pay the benefits in the future. To minimize that risk, employees often insist that the employer place the value of the deferred compensation into a "rabbi" trust, so named because the Internal Revenue Service ruled favorably on a deferred compensation arrangement created for a rabbi by his congregation (I.R.S. Priv. Ltr. Rul. 81-13-107 [December 31, 1980]). Using a rabbi trust, the employer funds a trust for the benefit of an employee, who will receive the funds on retirement at a designated age. The employer is taxed on any earnings in the trust prior to it being paid to the employee, and the assets of the trust must be available to satisfy the claims of the employer's general creditors before the deferred compensation due the employee is paid.

Welfare Benefit Plans

Employers often offer benefits such as health insurance, postretirement health insurance, life insurance, and other forms of noncash compensation. Known as welfare benefit plans, they are governed by ERISA and are a tax-free benefit for the employees (29 U.S.C. §1002[1]). Employers are not required to offer welfare benefits and can reserve the right to cancel them at any time (absent a collective bargaining agreement). As a result, employees and retirees are not assured that in the future they will receive welfare benefits currently provided by the plan.

One common welfare benefit provided by employers for older, retired employees is health care insurance. Many plans provide supplemental retiree health care benefits for those age 65 or older to cover co-pays, deductibles, and exclusions not covered by Medicare. The plan may also pay the monthly Medicare Part B premium. Unless prohibited by a collective bargaining agreement, the employer will almost certainly have reserved the right in the plan to amend or terminate such retiree health care benefits.

In light of the sharp increase in health care costs, many employers have reduced health care benefits for future retirees and in some cases even for those already retired. Retirement benefits based on a contractual obligation may not be unilaterally discontinued by the former employer. If, for example, Chi Company promised its employees that if they retired early, they would receive lifetime health care benefits, Chi Company will not be able to reduce benefits to those early retirees. It could, however, reduce benefits for future retirees.

Self-Employed Pension Plans (Keoghs)

Self-employed individuals can establish qualified pension plans, commonly known as Keogh or HR-10 plans (I.R.C. §401[c][1]). As with any qualified plan, contributions are tax deductible and distributions from the plan are included in the recipient's income. The earnings on the plan funds are not taxed until distributed.

Under the Internal Revenue Code, you are a self-employed individual if you earn income other than as an employee. You can be both an employee and a self-employed person. For example, Meredith is a lawyer employed by Gamma Inc. In her spare time she is self-employed as a dog breeder. With her earnings from the part-time self-employment, she can fund a Keogh retirement plan even if she also participates in the Gamma Inc. retirement plan.

Also available is the SEP, or simplified employee pension, which can be used by employers or self-employed persons to put up to15 percent of compensation into an IRA (I.R.C. §408[k]). The contribution to the SEP IRA is deductible, but all distributions from the account are taxable. An employee is fully vested in the SEP at all times.

Individual Retirement Accounts

To encourage individuals to save for their retirement, Congress created IRAs (I.R.C. §408). Some can be funded with tax-deductible dollars, but the distributions are subject to income tax; others are not deductible when funded, but the earnings on the account are never taxed; and still others are nondeductible when funded, and the investment earnings are taxed only when distributed (I.R.C. §2190).[1]

Some individuals are eligible to contribute and deduct up to $5,000 for contributions to an IRA if they are not an active participant in a qualified pension plan. Even individuals who are active participants in a qualified plan, or whose spouse is an active participant, may still qualify for deductible contributions to an IRA if their adjusted gross income falls below limits set by the Internal Revenue Code. No deductible contributions can be made to an IRA by an individual who reached age 70½ before the end of the taxable year. Individuals who are participants in retirement plans and whose income exceeds the limits for making deductible contributions may make nondeductible IRA contributions up to $3,000 annually.

The earnings on the IRA accumulate tax free until distribution and can be invested in many ways, including stocks, saving accounts, mutual funds, and bonds. However, the IRA cannot be invested in life insurance or collectibles such as stamps or art. All distributions from a deductible IRA are taxable on receipt. Distributions before age 59½ are subject to an additional 10 percent penalty tax except in the case of death, disability, or the distribution being paid subject to a divorce decree. The penalty also is not applicable if the distribution reimburses the participant, or the participant's spouse, child, or grandchild, for higher education expenses. Likewise, the penalty does not apply to distributions up to $10,000 per year for the expenses of a first-time home buyer, including the participant, his or her spouse, child, grandchild, or ancestor.

In contrast with the traditional IRA, a Roth IRA offers tax-free distributions, but the contributions to the IRA are not deductible from income. Because all distributions from a Roth IRA are tax free, the income earned on the Roth IRA account is never taxed (I.R.C. §408A). Individuals who do not participate in a qualified retirement plan are eligible to contribute to a Roth IRA without regard to their income. Individuals who do participate in a qualified retirement plan must have adjusted taxable income below certain phaseout amounts in order to participate.

The maximum annual contribution to a Roth IRA is the *lesser* of the amount of the individual's compensation reduced by any other IRA contribution or $5,000 in 2008. This amount will be increased annually for the cost of living. Individuals who are age 50 or older can contribute $6,000 (increased annually for the cost of living).

In addition to the annual contributions, individuals who have terminated employment with an employer who operates a defined contribution plan or 401(k) plan may roll over amounts from those accounts into an existing or new IRA. Such rollovers, if done according to Internal Revenue Code requirements, are not taxable. Individuals may also convert non-Roth IRAs into Roth IRAs subject to certain limits based on their adjusted taxable income. The conversion must be made within sixty days of receipt of any lump-sum distribution from the previous employer's plan.

Distributions from an IRA can be made any time after the contributor reaches age 59½ without regard to whether the individual recipient is retired. Except in the case of a Roth IRA, distributions must begin no later than April 1 following the calendar year in which the contributor reaches age 70½. The amount of the minimum mandatory distribution is determined using tables published by the Internal Revenue Service. If all of the amounts contributed to the IRA were deductible from income, all the distributions are taxable. Amounts that were not deducted when placed in the IRA are not taxable when distributed. The recipient is responsible for paying any income taxes due on distribution. This is true whether the recipient is the original contributor or the IRA beneficiary of a contributor who has died. For a Roth IRA, no distributions are taxed if made after the contributor turns age 59½ and no earlier than five years after the first day of the year in which a contribution was first made to a Roth IRA.

If the creator of an IRA dies before retiring or withdrawing all of the funds in the IRA account, the account passes to a named beneficiary. An IRA is not governed by the contributor's will, but by the beneficiary designation in the IRA agreement. It is therefore very important to select an IRA beneficiary when the account is established and to keep the beneficiary designation current in the event of changing circumstances such as divorce or death of a named beneficiary.

An IRA can be used to defer distributions for a considerable number of years. If the IRA recipient delays taking funds until age 70½ (the latest age to which distributions can be deferred), it is possible that the recipient will die before depleting the account. A spouse who is an IRA beneficiary can roll over the remaining IRA balance into the spouse's own IRA and distribute the funds over a lengthy payout period. If any other individual is designated as the beneficiary, that individual's life expectancy may be used to calculate the minimum distribution period. Even if a trust is named the beneficiary of the IRA, an extended payout will be permitted if the beneficiaries of the trust can be identified. They, in turn, will be treated as the designated beneficiaries who are eligible for extended payout treatment.

If the original IRA recipient dies before age 70½, all of the account must be paid out within five years unless the designated beneficiary is the spouse. A spousal beneficiary has the right to take minimum distributions calculated with reference to his or her life expectancy. Distributions to the surviving spouse need not begin until the date that the original IRA recipient would have turned age 70½.

Note

1. See IRS Publication 590 for detailed information about the operation and tax treatment of IRAs as well as current dollar amounts.

For More Information

U.S. Department of Labor
(http://www.dol.gov)

Follow the links for "frequently asked questions" to learn more about retirement plans and benefits.

5
Medicare

Did You Know?

- You are not eligible for Medicare until age 65 even if you receive Social Security retirement benefits earlier.
- Your Medicare Part A deductible is based on a "spell of illness" rather than on the calendar year.
- If you fail to enroll in Medicare Part B or Part D when you are first eligible, you may have to pay higher premiums.
- You cannot be denied a Medigap policy so long as you apply during the first six months after enrollment in Medicare.
- If you have health insurance through your employer or that of your spouse, you can delay Medicare Part B enrollment without penalty.
- If you have adequate prescription drug coverage through your employer or that of your spouse, you can delay enrollment in Part D without penalty.

A common misconception among the young is that Medicare is free government health insurance for seniors. Even though it is true that Medicare is available to individuals age 65 or older without regard to health status or financial resources, Medicare is not free. Medicare is part of the Social Security system and is funded through a combination of payroll taxes and general tax revenues, as well as the premiums, deductibles, and co-payments paid by participants.

This chapter discusses Medicare coverage, eligibility requirements, the costs, and participant rights. The discussion is organized according to the four parts of Medicare: Part A, which pays for hospitalization and other institutionalized care; Part B, which pays for physician charges and outpatient services; Medicare Advantage, or MA (formerly known as Part C or Medicare +

Choice), which provides health care through managed care companies; and Part D, which pays for prescription drugs. Medigap insurance, which is additional insurance that can be purchased to pay for costs not fully covered by Medicare, is also discussed.

Medicare Part A

Financing
A special federal wage tax funds most of Medicare Part A. Employees and employers each pay a 1.45 percent tax on employees' wages. Unlike the Social Security wage tax, there is no limit on the amount of wages subject to the Medicare wage tax. For example, Alice is employed by Acme Co. and earns $200,000 a year. Both Alice and Acme Co. will pay a Medicare wage tax of $2,900, or a combined tax of $5,800. Medicare Part A is also funded by the deductibles and co-payments paid by those who receive Medicare-covered services.

Eligibility and Enrollment
You are eligible for Medicare Part A without charge if you are age 65 or older and also eligible for Social Security old-age benefits or Railroad Retirement benefits, though you need not actually be collecting those benefits to enroll in Medicare (42 C.F.R. §406.10). Because there is no premium for Part A if you satisfy the work record eligibility requirements, you should enroll at age 65 even if you have other insurance. If you choose to receive Social Security old-age benefits before age 65, keep in mind that Medicare eligibility still does not begin until age 65.

Spouses, widows, or widowers of someone eligible for Social Security benefits are also entitled to Medicare Part A coverage when they reach age 65 (42 C.F.R. §406.10; 20 C.F.R. §§404.330, 404.335). A divorced spouse who has not remarried may be eligible for Medicare at age 65 based on the former spouse's eligibility if the marriage lasted at least ten years (42 C.F.R. §406.10; 20 C.F.R. §404.331).

Certain workers who meet the age 65 requirement are entitled to Medicare even though their employment was not covered by Social Security. This group includes federal, state, and local government employees hired after March 31, 1986, who did not participate in Social Security but paid the Medicare wage tax (42 C.F.R. §406.15).

If you are age 65 or older and receive Social Security (or Railroad Retirement) benefits, you are automatically enrolled in Medicare Part A. No separate application procedure is required. Individuals who are not receiving Social Security or Railroad Retirement benefits, but who are eligible for Medicare coverage, must apply for coverage to begin. You should file your application for Medicare during your initial enrollment period, which runs for seven months beginning three months before the month you turn age 65.

If you are over the age of 65 but do not qualify for Medicare Part A based on your work record (or that of your spouse), you can choose to enroll and pay a monthly premium (42 U.S.C. §1395i-2). To be eligible for voluntary enrollment, you must reside in the United States as a U.S. citizen or as a resident alien who has lived in the United States for the preceding five years. The amount of your premium will depend on how many work quarters you have paid Medicare wage tax, if any. In 2010 the maximum monthly premium amount was $461. The amount of the premium is adjusted annually.

Individuals who must pay the monthly Part A premium but who do not enroll during the initial enrollment period may do so during the general enrollment period from January 1 to March 31 each year. However, they will have to pay a 10 percent surcharge on the monthly premium for failure to enroll during the initial enrollment period. The surcharge lasts two years for every twelve months that enrollment was delayed (42 U.S.C. §1395i-2[c][6]).

If you are eligible for Medicare but have group health coverage through your employer or that of your spouse, you are entitled to a delayed eight-month enrollment period that begins on the first day of the month you are no longer covered by the employer-provided insurance (42 U.S.C. §1395i-2[c][7]). Thus, when your employer-provided insurance ends, you do not have to wait for a general enrollment period to enroll in Part A and Part B, and you will not be penalized for having delayed your enrollment past age 65.

In limited circumstances, individuals who are younger than age 65 may qualify for Medicare. Early eligibility is available for disabled individuals who have received Social Security disability payments for at least twenty-four months as well as for individuals with end-stage renal disease, which means irreversible kidney impairment that requires dialysis or kidney transplantation (42 C.F.R. §§406.12, 406.13).

Coverage

Medicare Part A reimburses the costs of hospital care, short-term skilled nursing facility care, part-time home health care after a stay in a hospital or nursing home, and most hospice care (42 U.S.C. §1395d). Medicare will reimburse the cost of only those services that are considered "reasonable and necessary" for the diagnosis or treatment of illness or injury. Procedures considered experimental and medically unproven are not covered by Medicare (42 U.S.C. §1395y[a]).

Hospitalization Benefits. Hospital inpatient benefits under Medicare Part A include reimbursement for daily hospital bed and board charges, nursing services, intern or residents-in-training services, medical social services, drugs, equipment, supplies, certain diagnostic and therapeutic services, and the cost of ambulance transportation to and from the hospital (42 C.F.R. §409.10[a]). Medicare will only pay the cost of a semiprivate hospital room.

If the beneficiary insists upon a private room, the hospital can charge the beneficiary the prevailing rate for the additional cost of a private room. If only private rooms are available, or a private room is medically necessary, the beneficiary will not be charged the extra cost. Part A does not pay for physicians (who are covered by Part B), nurse practitioners, private duty nurses or attendants (unless required by the beneficiary's condition), phones, televisions, or posthospitalization drugs, supplies, and equipment.

Part A beneficiaries must pay a deductible for the first sixty days of hospitalization in each spell of illness. This deductible, which was $1,100 in 2010, is adjusted annually. A spell of illness begins with admission to the hospital and ends when the patient has been out of the facility for a period of sixty consecutive days (42 U.S.C. §1395x[a]). If a patient is readmitted within the sixty days, even if for a different ailment, it will be considered within the same spell of illness. For example, Heather has a stroke and enters the hospital on May 1 but is discharged on May 21. She must pay the deductible. On June 15 Heather is readmitted to the hospital with pneumonia. Because she is within the same spell of illness, she does not have to pay the annual deductible upon her readmission to the hospital. Other than the deductible, Medicare Part A pays for all relevant services (excluding television and telephone expenses) during the first sixty days of a single spell of illness.

After the first sixty days of care in a single spell of illness, the beneficiary is responsible for a daily co-pay. In 2010, the co-pay was $275 a day. This co-pay continues for days sixty-one to ninety. After ninety days of coverage, the basic Medicare hospitalization insurance for that spell of illness ends. However, each Medicare Part A beneficiary has sixty lifetime reserve days of coverage. These sixty days are the maximum that each beneficiary receives and are not reset for subsequent spells of illness. Lifetime reserve days are also subject to a daily co-pay requirement, which was $550 in 2010. An individual can choose not to use his or her lifetime reserve by notifying the hospital in writing during the stay or within ninety days after discharge. For example, Julian has cancer and is admitted to the hospital on June 1. He remains in the hospital until September 10. The first ninety days (June 1 through August 29) are covered by Part A, though Julian has to pay the deductible and the daily co-pay. After August 29, he uses twelve of his sixty lifetime reserve days to cover the additional stay.

Medicare Part A has less generous benefits for inpatient psychiatric hospital care. Such care is subject to a lifetime maximum limit of 190 days. Once the beneficiary has been reimbursed for 190 days of care, no further reimbursement for inpatient care is available (42 U.S.C. §1395d[b][3]).

Skilled Nursing Facility Care. Medicare benefits for care in a skilled nursing facility (SNF), better known as a nursing home, are very limited. Part A reimburses only skilled nursing services, not custodial care, and will pay for only one hundred days of care for each spell of illness (42 U.S.C. §1395d[a][2]).

Four requirements must be met for SNF coverage under Part A. First, the facility must be Medicare approved, meet all federal and state standards, and have a transfer agreement with at least one hospital that participates in Medicare. Second, admission into a SNF must occur within thirty days after a discharge from a hospital; individuals who go directly from their homes to a SNF do not satisfy this requirement. Third, the preceding hospital stay must have lasted at least three days, not counting the day of discharge. Fourth, a medical professional must certify that the individual requires skilled nursing or skilled rehabilitative services that can be provided only in a SNF. This certification must show that the patient is receiving skilled care daily and that the care is for a condition that was treated in the hospital or related to that condition. In general, skilled nursing care involves services that require the skills of technical or professional personnel, including intravenous feedings, catheters, and injections (42 C.F.R. §409.33).

If all of the foregoing requirements are satisfied, Medicare Part A will pay the full cost of the first twenty days of SNF care for each spell of illness. The beneficiary must pay a daily co-pay for days twenty-one through one hundred, which was $137.50 in 2010. After the first one hundred days, Medicare pays no further costs for skilled nursing home care.

Home Health Care. Part A provides a limited range of home health services for individuals confined to their homes (42 U.S.C. §1395f[a][2][C]). To qualify, a beneficiary must be under a physician's care plan and confined to the home or to another residential living arrangement that is not a hospital or SNF (42 C.F.R. §409.42). The individual must need one or more of the following:

- intermittent skilled nursing care
- physical therapy
- speech-language pathology services
- continuing occupational therapy

This care must be furnished by a Medicare-certified home health care provider.

Medicare Part A home care is sometimes referred to as "postinstitutional care" because when an individual is enrolled in both Part A and Part B, Part A home care is available only after a three-consecutive-day hospital stay or posthospitalization extended care services in a SNF. Furthermore, the home health services must begin within fourteen days after the individual was discharged from the hospital or SNF (42 U.S.C. §1395x[tt][1]). Medicare Part A pays for home health care for one hundred visits within a "home health spell of illness" (42 U.S.C. §1395d[a][3]), which begins on the first day that the individual receives home health services and ends sixty days after the last day the individual receives home health services or was not a patient in a hospital or SNF (42 U.S.C. §1395x[tt][2]). If the foregoing requirements for home health services under Part A are not met, the individual may be eligible for home health services under Medicare Part B. Part B generally provides limited home care benefits when a homebound beneficiary has exhausted the maximum one hundred visits under Part A, does not meet the prior institutional care requirement, or has only Part B coverage.

Only Medicare beneficiaries who are confined to the home, or are "homebound," are eligible for Medicare home health care. An individual is homebound if leaving home takes a considerable or taxing effort. Examples include individuals confined to a wheelchair or who require the aid of crutches to walk, those who have lost the use of upper extremities and require assistance to open doors or use stairways, and individuals who, because of dementia or blindness, require the assistance of another to leave the house. An individual who meets the definition of homebound but does in fact leave home infrequently for nonmedical reasons (such as a trip for religious services) still qualifies for home health services. In addition, individuals who attend adult day care are eligible for home health care if they are otherwise homebound (42 U.S.C. §1395f[a]).

Covered services include physical, occupational, and speech therapy; medical supplies; and durable medical equipment. The nursing care must be reasonable and necessary as well as part time or intermittent, which is defined as care provided less than seven days each week or less than eight hours a day over a period of not more than twenty-one days. The total care each week cannot exceed twenty-eight hours, though it can be as much as thirty-five hours if determined to be necessary on a case-by-case basis (42 U.S.C. §1395x[m]).

Care may be provided by more than one provider. For example, a nurse might provide care for one hour a day, five days a week, and a physical therapist might visit three days a week for one hour. The hour and day limits may be extended in exceptional circumstances if the attending physician can predict when the need for such care will end. In other words, home health care will not provide assistance for an indefinite period.

Part A does not cover drugs, delivered meals, and homemaker services. However, for the services covered, Medicare will pay 100 percent of the cost, except for durable medical equipment for which the patient must pay 20 percent. Supplemental medical insurance may cover this portion of the cost.

Hospice Care. Hospice care is a combination of home care, occasional inpatient institutionalization, and palliative care (care for pain control and comfort) (42 U.S.C. §1395x[dd][1]). To qualify for Part A hospice care, a patient must be certified as not likely to live more than six months. Hospice care is meant to provide pain relief and symptom control, rather than curative treatment for the patient's condition. The goal of hospice care is to improve the quality of the patient's remaining life by reducing pain, stress, and anxiety. Hospice care is usually delivered in the patient's home or a homelike setting and generally consists of nursing and attendant care that supplements family caregiving.

Patients must elect to receive hospice care instead of other Medicare services. In other words, the patient must be willing to discontinue attempts to cure the medical condition. The patient is initially entitled to ninety days of hospice care but can continue to receive services if the hospice medical director or the patient's physician certifies continued eligibility. At any time, the patient can revoke hospice care and return to full Part A benefits (43 C.F.R. §418.28[a]).

Generally, Part A will pay for all costs associated with hospice care, including registered nursing care, therapy, homemaker services, and counseling. The two exceptions to full coverage are prescription drugs and respite care. Patients in hospice care must pay the lesser of 5 percent of the cost of outpatient drugs or $5 per prescription. They must also pay 5 percent of the Medicare reimbursement rate for respite care, which is short-term institutionalization of a patient in order to give the regular caregiver a break from his or her duties.

Payment Procedures
Medicare does not directly pay hospitals, doctors, or other health care providers. Instead, Medicare contracts with large, private insurance companies that reimburse providers for covered services. Medicare in turn reimburses the insurance companies. The provider generally takes care of the paperwork and bills the patient for the deductible or co-pay. The provider may also appeal a decision of Medicare not to reimburse certain treatment for a patient.

If a Medicare beneficiary has been admitted to the hospital, but the attending physician and the hospital agree that the stay will not be reimbursed by Medicare, they must promptly notify the patient of their opinion. Having notified the patient of noncoverage, the hospital can begin to charge the patient for the customary cost of care beginning on the third day after the notification. The patient has the option of paying for the care or appealing the decision.

Appeals from Denial of Coverage
Medicare Part A will pay only for medical care that is "medically reasonable and necessary." This vague term sometimes is misinterpreted by providers that mistakenly believe Medicare will pay for the care provided. Patients are not financially responsible for such care if the patient did not know or could not have been expected to know that Medicare would refuse to pay for the

services. The provider will usually be responsible for the cost of care if the patient was not notified in advance of Medicare noncoverage.

If the provider properly informs the patient that Medicare will not pay for medical care and Medicare refuses to pay, the patient can request a reconsideration of the denied coverage within sixty days of receiving the original decision. Further appeal is allowed within sixty days of receiving the reconsideration decision if the amount in question is at least $100. This appeal takes place before an administrative law judge. Finally, the decision of the administrative law judge can be appealed to a federal court if the case involves more than $1,000 (42 U.S.C. §1395ff[b]; 42 C.F.R. §478). If the initial denial was made by a state quality improvement organization (QIO), the dollar amounts are $200 and $2000, respectively (42 C.F.R. §§478.40, 478.46).

Typically, it is the provider that appeals a denied coverage decision because it is the provider that is at financial risk if the cost of care is not paid. To avoid coverage disputes, hospitals rely on utilization review committees to determine for what and how much Medicare will pay. If the patient's physician who requested the treatment disagrees with the utilization review committee, the hospital can appeal to the state QIO. The QIO will determine if the proposed care is medically necessary and eligible for Medicare coverage.

Patients can appeal Medicare coverage decisions to the QIO as well. For example, a patient who does not believe he or she should be discharged from the hospital can appeal to the QIO and will not be charged until the appeal is approved or denied. If the patient wishes to contest the bill, an administrative appeal can be made within 120 days if the claim exceeds $200 (42 C.F.R.§478.46). A patient can appeal to a federal court if the claim exceeds $2,000 (42 U.S.C. §1395ff).

Many patient appeals arise when a hospital wishes to discharge the patient to a SNF, but the patient objects because either there is no Medicare skilled nursing home bed available or no bed is available in a facility acceptable to the patient. A hospital cannot discharge a patient in need of skilled nursing care unless there is an available Medicare skilled nursing home bed. If a skilled nursing home bed is available, Medicare will not pay for additional days in the hospital even though the patient refuses to transfer. Although the law does not provide a right to refuse a transfer to a Medicare skilled nursing home bed, a patient who appeals the discharge decision to the state QIO may gain a few extra covered days in which to arrange more satisfactory posthospitalization care.

Medicare Part B

Financing
Medicare Part B, Supplemental Medical Insurance, is voluntary medical insurance that helps pay the costs of physician and outpatient services (42

U.S.C. §1395j). Participants in Medicare Part B must pay monthly premiums that vary according to the participant's income—the higher the income, the higher the premium. Premiums are set at a level so that in the aggregate they cover approximately 25 percent of the cost of Part B, with general federal revenues paying the rest. The premium is deducted from the beneficiary's monthly Social Security payment or other government benefit payment. If a beneficiary receives no government benefit payments, the premium is billed monthly.

The basic monthly premium in 2010 was $96.40 for individuals with a modified adjusted gross income (AGI) of $85,000 or less and for couples with a modified AGI of $170,000 or less.[1] For purposes of this computation, your modified AGI is your adjusted gross (taxable) income plus tax-exempt interest income. Table 5.1 shows the respective premium levels for individuals and couples who had modified AGI above the standard premium levels in 2010. Medicare Part B premium rates are adjusted annually.

Eligibility and Enrollment

Eligibility for Part B is the same as for Part A, although all participants in Part B must pay a premium (see the Eligibility and Enrollment discussion for Medicare Part A). Individuals who receive Social Security or Railroad Retirement benefits and who are at least 65 years old are enrolled automatically. However, automatically enrolled beneficiaries are notified of their right to decline Part B.

Individuals who are not entitled to premium-free Part A and who choose not to enroll in Part A may still enroll in Part B. The enrollment period begins three months before the month that the individual turns age 65 and continues for seven months. An individual who delays enrollment beyond this initial enrollment period may enroll during the general enrollment period from January 1 to March 31 each year, but he or she will have to pay a 10 percent surcharge on the monthly premium.

Table 5.1   2010 Medicare Part B Premium Rates

	Modified AGI	Monthly Premium
Individuals	$85,001–107,000	$154.70
Couple	$170,001–214,000	$154.70
Individuals	$107,001–160,000	$221.00
Couples	$214,001–320,000	$221.00
Individuals	$160,001–214,000	$287.30
Couples	$320,001–428,000	$287.30
Individuals	Above $214,000	$353.60
Couples	Above $428,000	$353.60

Like the surcharge for delayed premium-paid Part A enrollment, the surcharge for delayed Part B enrollment lasts two years for every twelve months that enrollment is delayed (42 U.S.C. §1395i-2[c][6]; 42 C.R.F. §408.22). However, this increase does not apply to those who delay enrollment because they have employer-provided health insurance from their own employment or that of a spouse. These individuals have a special eight-month enrollment period that begins when their employer-provided health insurance ends (42 U.S.C. §1395i-2[c][7]).

Coverage
Medicare Part B reimburses physicians' services, including those provided in a hospital (42 U.S.C. §1395k[a]; 42 C.F.R. §410.10). Part B also covers diagnostic services, outpatient therapy, durable medical equipment, ambulance services, medical supplies, dialysis, pacemakers, blood transfusions, and pneumococcal and hepatitis B vaccines. There are limitations, however, on these covered services. For example, covered ambulance service is limited to transportation from home to a hospital or SNF and only if it is medically necessary because any other form of transportation could harm the patient. Outpatient therapy is subject to a billing cap and is covered only if prescribed by a physician. A doctor's prescription is also required for durable medical equipment.

Among the services that Part B does *not* cover are routine physical examinations, dental care, custodial care, routine foot care (unless necessary for an underlying condition), cosmetic surgery, and eye examinations. Also, Part B does not cover eyeglasses and contact lenses (except for postsurgical devices), hearing aids, orthopedic shoes (unless they are a part of leg braces), and personal comfort items in a hospital.

Payment Procedures
The beneficiary must pay an annual deductible for Part B, which in 2010 was $155. The beneficiary is also responsible for a 20 percent co-pay for most doctor services, outpatient therapy, preventive services, and durable medical equipment. Medicare Part B reimbursement is limited to what are known as approved charges. For each service, Medicare establishes an approved charge, which is the amount that Medicare believes appropriate for that procedure. Medicare then pays for 80 percent of the approved charge, regardless of the amount charged by the physician (42 U.S.C.§1395l[a]). The other 20 percent is paid by the patient.

Physicians often find collecting patient payments costly and sometimes impossible. To assist physicians, Medicare permits them to "participate" in Part B. This is sometimes known as "taking assignment" and means that the physician agrees not to charge the patient more than the Medicare-approved charge. In return, Medicare directly reimburses the physician for its 80 percent obligation. In some states, physicians are required by law to participate in Medicare as a condition of their licensure. In most states, physicians need not participate. Physicians who do not participate must collect the entire 100 percent from the patient, who in turn is reimbursed by Medicare for its 80 percent payment obligation.

A physician who does not participate in Medicare is allowed to charge the patient up to 15 percent more than the Medicare-approved charge. The patient is responsible for the 20 percent co-payment, plus the extra 15 percent of the Medicare-approved charge. For example, Dr. Jones does not participate in Medicare Part B. Andy visits Dr. Jones and receives care for which Medicare Part B has established an approved charge of $1,000. Dr. Jones can charge Andy $1,150. Medicare is obligated to pay $800 (80% × $1,000, which is the approved charge). Andy will pay $1,150, which includes the 20 percent co-pay of the approved charge ($200), the additional 15 percent ($150), and the $800 that will be reimbursed eventually by Medicare.

Medicare Part B pays 100 percent of certain clinical laboratory services, vaccines, and home health services. However, Part B pays only 50 percent of the approved physician's charges for outpatient treatment for mental, psychoneurotic, and personality disorders (42 C.F.R. §410.152).

Appeals from Denial of Coverage
Part B claims are handled on Medicare's behalf by private insurance companies called "carriers." The patient can request that a denied claim be reconsidered by the carrier within six months of the date of the denial. If not satisfied, a patient can appeal to the carrier's hearing officer within six months of the reconsidered decision. This option is available only if the dispute is for more than $100, though claims can be combined to meet the minimum amount (42 C.F.R. §405.815). Appeals from the hearing officer go before an administrative law judge if filed within sixty days of the hearing officer's decision and worth at least $500, either alone or in combination with other claims. Cases involving more than $1,000 can be appealed to the federal court system.

Medicare Advantage

Medicare Advantage (formerly known as Medicare Part C or Medicare + Choice) is a managed care alternative to the original fee-for-service Medicare (42 U.S.C. §1395w-22). Seniors may elect to enroll in MA instead of participating in Medicare Parts A and B. Although MA plans must provide all Part A and Part B covered services, most provide additional coverage as an incentive for seniors to join.

MA plans vary, so if you are considering MA, you should read the plan materials carefully. Often MA plans charge a single monthly premium that covers Part A and Part B services, Medicare Part D prescription drugs, and sometimes extra services, such as vision, hearing, and dental, that are not covered by original Medicare. However, with some MA plans, you must still pay all or part of your Part B premium. Co-payments and deductibles also vary by plan.

If you choose to enroll in MA, you will not need a Medigap supplemental insurance policy. In fact, Medigap insurance does not cover MA plan deductibles and co-payments. One risk of enrolling in MA and dropping your Medigap policy is that you may not be able to obtain another Medigap policy if you later decide to return to original Medicare. However, there are protections for individuals who join MA for the first time and who decide to return to original Medicare within the first twelve months. Generally, these individuals are entitled to be reinstated under their former Medigap policy provided that the company still offers it.

MA plans appear in several forms, including health maintenance organizations (HMOs), preferred provider organizations (PPOs), provider-sponsored organizations (PSOs), medical savings account plans (MSAs), private fee-for-service plans (PFFSs), and special needs plans (SNPs). The rules for each type of MA plan differ significantly. For example, whether you need to choose a primary care doctor or must obtain a referral to see a specialist depends on the plan. Under some plans, if you use out-of-network providers, you may have to pay a higher cost, or, in some cases, the full cost of services received. Before you enroll in an MA plan, be sure you understand what it provides and how it operates.

Eligibility and Enrollment

If you are eligible for Medicare Part A or Part B, you are eligible to enroll in an MA plan. You can elect to enroll during an initial eligibility period that runs from three months before you turn age 65 and continues for seven months. You can also enroll in, change, or drop your MA plan each year between November 15 and December 31, with your new coverage beginning on January 1 of the following year. Changes during the general Medicare enrollment period between January 1 and March 31 are prohibited if the MA plan is an MSA or involves prescription drug coverage.

Generally, MA participants must stay enrolled for the calendar year in which MA coverage begins. You may be able to join, change, or drop an MA plan at times other than the usual enrollment periods if you live in an institution, qualify for a subsidy to help pay Medicare prescription drug costs, are qualified for both Medicare and Medicaid, or move out of your plan's service area.

Coverage

MA plans must offer the same benefits as Part A and Part B, but to encourage enrollment, they typically offer additional benefits, such as routine physical examinations, eyeglasses, hearing aids, and dental care (42 U.S.C.

§1395mm[c]). Many offer better prescription drug subsidies than Medicare Part D. The extent and value of the benefits offered depend primarily on the amount of the reimbursement provided to the plans by Medicare. Therefore, the greater the payment by Medicare is to the plan for each Medicare enrollee, the more generous the plan can be in the provision of benefits. Because Congress periodically changes the amount of the MA plan subsidies, the number of such plans and the benefits also periodically change.

Appeals from Denial of Coverage
MA plans are required to provide dispute resolution procedures. The plan must also provide written notice of denial of services or termination of hospitalization and must offer beneficiaries a form of internal review. The beneficiary must be given sixty days to request a review of a contested care decision as well as an expedited form of review.

Medicare Part D

The Medicare Prescription Drug Improvement and Modernization Act of 2003 added prescription drug coverage known as Medicare Part D (42 U.S.C. §1395w-101). Part D subsidizes prescription drug costs by providing financial assistance to private drug plans (PDPs) that sell prescription drug insurance to individuals eligible for or enrolled in Medicare Part A or Part B. Individuals enrolled in Medicare Advantage generally receive prescription drug assistance though their MA plan.

Eligibility and Enrollment
Anyone eligible for or enrolled in either Part A or Part B is eligible to enroll in Part D. Enrollment is voluntary. Beneficiaries enroll by joining one of the federally subsidized prescription drug plans offered by private insurance companies. The beneficiary pays a monthly insurance premium to the plan insurer. The plans vary greatly in coverage as well as in the specific drugs that are available on the plan drug list known as the "formulary." The formulary may contain different tiers or categories of drugs that have different costs.

The monthly premiums in 2010 averaged a little less than $39 and ranged nationally from $8.80 to $120.20, depending on the amount of coverage and the formulary. Although plans cannot refuse to enroll Medicare beneficiaries, they can and do charge higher premiums in geographical areas where residents have higher drug expenses. Low-income enrollees, as well as those eligible for both Medicare and Medicaid, or SSI, are eligible for a reduction in cost or a complete subsidy.

Enrollment in Part D occurs during the coordinated annual enrollment election period that runs each year from November 15 through December

31. Beneficiaries who move or have other reasons for a special enrollment period are accommodated as necessary. Individuals eligible for both Medicare and Medicaid are automatically enrolled as soon as their eligibility for Part D is determined. After enrollment, those beneficiaries have the right to opt out.

An individual who fails to enroll when first eligible is subject to a late enrollment penalty in the form of increased premiums unless the individual has comparable prescription drug coverage (known as "creditable coverage") and is not without such coverage for more than sixty-three days prior to enrollment (42 C.F.R. §423.46). Typically, this includes individuals whose employer provides them with health insurance. Those who do not enroll in the program when they initially become eligible must pay a penalty of 1 percent of the national average premium for *each* month that they delay enrollment unless they had creditable coverage. This penalty applies as long as the beneficiary is enrolled in Medicare Part D.

In lieu of enrolling in a PDP, beneficiaries can join a Medicare Advantage plan that offers prescription drug coverage. MA plan prescription drug coverage is comparable to or better than the coverage required by Medicare Part D. Beneficiaries do not have to enroll in any form of Part D if they choose not to participate.

Coverage

Participating plans cannot require Part D beneficiaries to pay more than federally established deductibles. Most offer more generous terms. In 2010, a plan could not require an annual deductible of more than $310. The deductible is adjusted each year to reflect the annual growth in the spending by beneficiaries on Part D drugs. After the deductible is met, in 2010 the beneficiary could be required to pay 25 percent of the drug costs incurred between $310 and $2,830. The beneficiary could then be required to pay 100 percent of prescription drug costs from $2,830 to $6,440. This amount is known as the "donut hole" in the plan coverage. Once the beneficiary has reached the other side of the donut hole ($6,440 in 2010), he or she is eligible for catastrophic coverage under which the beneficiary pays the greater of 5 percent of the cost of the prescription or $2.50 for generic drugs and $6.30 for brand name drugs. Institutionalized beneficiaries, such as those in a nursing home, have no such co-pay.

As a result of the foregoing drug coverage structure, a Part D beneficiary in 2010 could be required to pay as much as $4,550 in drug costs before achieving catastrophic coverage. For example, Lucas enrolls in a prescription drug plan that uses the maximum deductible and co-pays allowed by law. Table 5.2 lists the costs he will incur. If Lucas has any additional drug costs in the plan year, he will qualify for catastrophic coverage.

Note that Lucas may elect to join a plan that does not require him to pay all of the deductible, the 25 percent co-pay, or even all of the costs of the donut hole (the uncovered costs between $2,830 and $6,440). Most plans

Table 5.2   2010 Medicare Part D Out-of-Pocket Costs

Deductible	$310
25% of costs between $310 deductible and $2,830	$630
100% of costs between $2,830 and $6,440	$3,610
Total out-of-pocket cost	$4,550

provide some relief from the maximum participation amounts that can be charged to beneficiaries, but many do not provide any coverage of the donut hole. However, beneficiaries can expect higher premiums the greater the plan coverage and the lower the costs-per-prescription paid by the beneficiary.

Part D covers only prescription drugs and only those that are considered reasonable and necessary. Vaccines not covered by Part B are covered by Part D. Otherwise, Part D will not pay for a drug if either Part A or Part B will pay for it. Plans may also exclude drugs that are excluded under Medicaid, such as vitamins, barbiturates, and those for weight loss, fertility, cosmetic results, and cough or cold relief.

PDPs may limit drug coverage to a set list of drugs created by the secretary of the Department of Health and Human Services (HHS) or may design other lists subject to approval by the secretary of HHS. PDPs are prohibited, however, from designing lists with the purpose of excluding beneficiary groups with certain drug needs. PDPs may change their lists of covered drugs annually, but they must provide notice to the plan beneficiaries.

MA plans may offer coverage as an alternative to Part D if the coverage has an equal value to Part D plans and is approved by the secretary of HHS. As of January 1, 2006, companies offering Medigap insurance could no longer sell new policies with prescription drug coverage.

Appeals from Denial of Coverage

PDPs are required to establish a process for handling beneficiary grievances. Although PDP coverage is defined by set lists of prescription drugs, the plans must provide access at a favorable price to all medically necessary drugs not on the list. If unsatisfied with the coverage, a beneficiary can appeal a denial of coverage determination. Appeals under Part D are first subject to internal review by the PDP. An unfavorable decision for the beneficiary can be appealed to an independent review entity for reconsideration. The appeal next goes to a hearing before an administrative law judge. A beneficiary can appeal further to the Medicare Appeals Council and finally to a federal district court.

Medigap Insurance Policies

Medicare does not provide complete coverage to its beneficiaries, who must pay deductibles, co-pays, coinsurance, and the cost of noncovered services.

The out-of-pocket amount that any beneficiary will have to pay is difficult to estimate in advance, but it can be considerable. As a result, many individuals purchase supplemental Medicare health care insurance known as Medigap because it fills in the coverage "gaps" left by Medicare. These insurance policies are sold by private insurance companies and are entirely optional.

As of 2009, federal standards for Medigap policies limited all policies to one of twelve standard packages of coverage identified in most states by the letters A through L, with A being the least comprehensive (42 U.S.C. §1395ss). As of June 1, 2010, plans E, H, I, and J will be phased out and two new plans—M and N—will be available. In some states, another Medigap alternative called Medicare SELECT will be offered. Medicare SELECT policies require participants to use designated hospitals and doctors to get full coverage. All packages with the same letter designation are identical across all insurance companies, although the premium may vary from company to company.

Insurance companies do not have to offer all Medigap packages and can restrict availability of plans to certain groups based on factors such as age or medical conditions. Because companies set their own premiums for the various packages, different companies charge different premiums for identical coverage. If you are thinking of buying a Medigap policy, consider the financial strength of the insurance company, the customer service offered, and how willing the company is to pay benefits.

Consumer Protection Provisions

Federal law provides several consumer protections for those who purchase Medigap insurance (42 U.S.C. §1395ss[o]). First, you may not be denied a policy because of a preexisting condition if you apply during the first six months after enrollment in Medicare. Second, your Medigap policy must be guaranteed renewable unless the premium is not paid or there was a material misrepresentation in the application. Third, insurance companies are prohibited from selling more than one Medigap policy to any one buyer. A company that violates this prohibition may face criminal penalties and the buyer will be refunded any premiums paid on the second plan. Every state has a State Health Insurance Assistance Program (SHIP) that provides free counseling about Medicare, Medigap, and PDPs.

Benefits

All Medigap plans within the A through J plan categories contain the following basic benefits:

- Medicare Part A daily hospitalization co-payment for days 61–90
- Medicare Part A daily lifetime reserve days co-payment
- an additional 365 days of hospitalization without any co-payment

- Medicare Part B 20 percent co-payment for medical services and durable medical equipment (after the annual deductible is met)
- the first three pints of blood not covered by Medicare

In addition, a hospice care co-insurance benefit will be added to all new Medigap policies beginning June 1, 2010.

The foregoing basic benefits are the only benefits included in a Medigap plan A policy. Plans B through J offer these benefits as well as some combination of the following benefits:

- Part A hospital inpatient deductible
- Part B deductible
- SNF co-insurance for days twenty-one to one hundred
- foreign travel emergency costs (subject to limit)
- some percentage of Part B excess charges

Prescription drug benefits are not available under new Medigap policies because of the availability of prescription drug coverage under Part D.

Medigap plans K and L differ from plans A through J in two primary ways—they have lower monthly premiums, and they have higher out-of-pocket costs. After the beneficiary meets the out-of-pocket limit and Part B deductible, these plans pay 100 percent of covered services for the rest of the year.

Medigap plans M and N also offer lower premiums in exchange for higher cost sharing. For example, participants in plan M must pay their own Part B deductible and half of the Part A deductible. Plan N participants cost share through co-payments rather than deductibles.

Costs

The cost of a Medigap policy depends not only on the coverage offered, but also on the way the policy is "rated." Policies are rated in three different ways: (1) based on the age of the beneficiary when the policy is issued, (2) adjusted annually based on the beneficiary's current age, or (3) set without regard to the beneficiary's age. Other factors that may affect the policy's cost include gender-based or smoking-status discounts, as well as a high-deductible option if available.

The Best Medicare Plan for You

Choices about original Medicare, Medicare Advantage, Medicare Part D, and Medigap insurance are complex and depend on your personal situation and preferences. Fortunately, many resources are available to help you make these decisions. SHIPs provide free one-on-one counseling about these choices. Medicare also makes available to all eligible beneficiaries a publication called *Medicare and You*, tailored for your state. This publication is available in print and online. It contains the phone number for your state's SHIP program as well as state-specific information about Medicare Advantage and Part D drug plans.

Note

1. Some persons will pay a slightly higher Part B basic premium of $110.50 if they are new enrollees or do not pay their premium through a deduction from Social Security benefits.

For More Information

Center for Medicare Advocacy (860-456-7790)
(http://www.medicareadvocacy.org)

Find specific information by topic about all aspects of Medicare coverage, proposed Medicare changes, and guidance for asserting your rights under Medicare.

Medicare (800-MEDICARE)
(http://www.medicare.gov)

Find information about all aspects of Medicare coverage and benefits including enrollment, choice of plans, costs, and appeals. Links are provided to state-specific resources.

National SHIP Resource Center
(http://www.shiptalk.org)

Find information about free one-on-one counseling to help you make decisions about Medicare and other health insurance matters.

6

Medicaid and Long-Term Care Insurance

Did You Know?

- Medicaid eligibility criteria vary from state to state.
- Medicaid may be available to pay for long-term care services in your home.
- Even if your spouse needs Medicaid nursing home benefits, you can maintain your lifestyle at home with careful advance planning.
- Gifts you make today could disqualify you or your spouse from Medicaid later.
- Special long-term care insurance may make it possible for you to keep your assets and still qualify for Medicaid.

Perhaps what seniors fear most is that someday they will need long-term care. Second to this fear is the worry about how they will pay for it. Although Medicaid is the single largest source of funding for nursing home care, not all seniors qualify for Medicaid.

If you do not meet Medicaid's financial eligibility requirements, you must rely on your own private funds or insurance to pay for your long-term care. Whether received in a nursing home, an assisted living facility, or at home, long-term care is expensive. This chapter discusses Medicaid long-term care benefits, eligibility requirements, and special planning considerations for married persons. Asset transfers that may cause you to lose Medicaid eligibility are also discussed.

In addition to Medicaid, long-term care insurance is explained. Long-term care insurance may be a good alternative if you cannot qualify for

Medicaid. It may also be beneficial if you could meet the Medicaid income requirements but have assets that exceed what Medicaid allows. Many states now permit qualified persons to both shelter assets and receive Medicaid if they first exhaust benefits from a state-approved long-term care insurance policy.

Medicaid Benefits

Medicaid is a federal program, but it is administered by the states. Medicaid pays the medical expenses of defined categories of persons who also meet financial eligibility requirements (42 U.S.C. §1396a). Medicaid categories of coverage include low-income children, pregnant women, adults in families with dependent children, and the aged, blind, and disabled. This chapter looks at Medicaid eligibility for persons who qualify because they are aged—that is, age 65 or older.

Every state as well as the District of Columbia participates in Medicaid. The federal government pays for about one-half of the cost of Medicaid-covered services, with the states paying the rest. In some states, the program is referred to as Medical Assistance (California labels it Medi-Cal). Regardless of the title, Medicaid pays almost one-half of all long-term care spending in the United States. One-third of Medicaid dollars are spent on health care for seniors.

Even though states must follow federal Medicaid standards, they may offer more liberal benefits than those required by federal law (42 U.S.C. §§1396a[a][10][A], 1396d[a]). The mandatory services that all states must provide include the following:

- inpatient and outpatient services
- laboratory and x-ray services
- physicians' services
- nursing facility services
- home health services for individuals who qualify for nursing facility care

Optional services include these services:

- care provided by licensed practitioners other than physicians
- diagnostic, screening, and preventive services
- physical, speech, occupational, and audiology therapies
- dentures, prosthetic devices, and eyeglasses
- case management
- durable medical equipment
- inpatient and nursing facility services in an institution for mental diseases

- hospice services
- transportation services
- home and community-based waiver services
- PACE services (Programs of All-Inclusive Care for the Elderly)

Although prescription drug coverage is an optional service, all states include some level of prescription drug coverage in their Medicaid plan.[1]

More than one-half of the total optional state Medicaid spending is for long-term care.[2] Of the Medicaid spending on long-term care, approximately two-thirds pays for institutional care, with the remaining one-third paying for home and community-based waiver services.[3] Unlike Medicare, which pays for only skilled nursing care on a limited basis, Medicaid covers both skilled and custodial nursing home care.

Given that the most costly aspect of Medicaid reimbursement is nursing home care, federal waivers permit states to cover less expensive long-term care provided in the home or community (42 U.S.C. §1396n[c]; 42 C.F.R. §440.180). Home and community-based services can include case management, homemaker services, home health aides, personal care services, adult day health services, respite care, and habilitation services (42 C.F.R. §440.180[b]). Although home care and community-based care are less expensive than nursing home care, the availability of waiver services usually results in an increased number of Medicaid applications. This is because home care is more attractive to most seniors than nursing home care.

Thus, even though the cost per Medicaid applicant may be less for home and community-based care than for nursing home care, the widespread availability of waiver services could substantially raise a state's Medicaid budget. Therefore, the federal government permits states to limit the number of waiver participants. In most states, there is a long waiting list for home and community-based services.

Medicaid Eligibility

Although federal law sets the basic parameters for Medicaid eligibility, state interpretations of the federal standards differ, resulting in eligibility standards that are not completely consistent from state to state. Another source of inconsistency among the states is something known as the 209(b) option. In 1972, Congress replaced other joint federal/state welfare programs with the Supplemental Security Income (SSI) program (see Chapter 3 for a discussion of SSI). Under SSI eligibility guidelines, an increased number of persons would have qualified for Medicaid. Fearing that states would exit the program, Congress allowed states to retain their pre-SSI Medicaid eligibility standards (Pub. L. No. 92-603, §209[b]; 42 U.S.C. §1396a[f]). Currently, eleven states utilize the 209(b) option to require tougher financial limits for

Medicaid eligibility. They are Connecticut, Hawaii, Illinois, Indiana, Minnesota, Missouri, New Hampshire, North Dakota, Ohio, Oklahoma, and Virginia.

Most seniors who qualify for Medicaid do so because they are considered "categorically needy"—in other words, they fall within the federal definition of aged (age 65 or older), blind, or disabled, and are eligible for SSI (42 U.S.C. §1396a). Although 209(b) states can use more restrictive Medicaid eligibility requirements than the SSI criteria, they must allow applicants who would otherwise qualify for Medicaid to "spend down" excess income. Applicants may deduct their medical expenses from their income to accomplish this spend-down (Pub. L. No. 92-603, §209[b]; 42 U.S.C. §1396a[f]).

States also have the option of extending Medicaid eligibility to individuals who are "medically needy" (42 U.S.C. §1396a[a][10][C]). More than two-thirds of states grant Medicaid to medically needy individuals. The definition of medically needy varies from state to state, as do the available benefits. In general, you are considered medically needy if you cannot afford the cost of your nursing home care, your assets are within SSI eligibility limits, but your income exceeds the SSI eligibility threshold. Medicaid will make up the shortfall when a medically needy applicant's monthly income is inadequate to cover the monthly nursing home bill.

All U.S. citizens and certain legal immigrants can qualify for Medicaid. Because Medicaid is administered at the state level, an applicant must also be considered a resident of that state. You are considered a resident of the state in which you live and intend to stay, permanently or indefinitely (42 C.F.R. §435.403[i][1][i]). Individuals over age 21 who are unable to express their intent are considered residents of the state where they are physically present (42 C.F.R. §435.403[i][3]). States cannot impose minimum residency requirements for Medicaid eligibility, such as a waiting period for persons moving into the state (42 C.F.R. §435.403[j]).

Consider the example of Sam, age 77, who lives in Arizona but has a stroke while visiting his daughter in Ohio. Due to the effects of the stroke, Sam moves into a nursing home in Ohio. Because he is physically present in Ohio, Sam will be entitled to Ohio Medicaid to help cover the costs of his nursing home care if he otherwise meets the eligibility requirements.

Resource and Income Requirements

At the heart of Medicaid eligibility are the resource and income requirements. These requirements vary depending on the state, the applicant's marital status, and, if married, whether one or both members of the couple are seeking Medicaid services in a nursing home. The following discussion is a general overview of Medicaid resource and income requirements. Special considerations for married persons are addressed in a subsequent section.

Resources

To qualify for Medicaid as categorically needy or medically needy, you must also meet the state's resource eligibility test. Most states use the SSI resource standard, but 209(b) states are permitted to use more restrictive standards (42 C.F.R. §435.840). If you live in a state that uses SSI resource limits and you are unmarried, you cannot have more than $2,000 in countable resources. If you are married, the countable resource limit is $3,000. Some states use slightly higher dollar amounts. By comparison, in Indiana (a 209[b] state) an individual may have only $1,500 in countable resources and a couple may have only $2,250.

Countable Resources. Most states use the SSI resource rules to define countable resources. Countable resources are any assets you own that count toward the Medicaid resource limit. The following are examples of assets that are generally considered countable:

- cash on hand (other than current income)
- financial accounts (such as bank accounts, certificates of deposit, individual retirement accounts, and Keogh plans)
- stocks and bonds
- assets in trust (but only to the extent the assets are available to you)

Like assets in trust, pension plan assets and annuities are countable resources only if you can access them. For example, if you have the ability to make lump-sum withdrawals from a pension plan or annuity, the assets are deemed available and countable, even if the withdrawal will trigger fees or penalties. Countable resources are valued at their fair market value, adjusted for any early withdrawal penalties or other legitimate fees.

Assets that were transferred for less than fair market value within sixty months of the date an applicant would otherwise be eligible for Medicaid are also treated as a countable resource.[4] Such transfers result in a penalty period of ineligibility (see the asset transfers discussion in this chapter). Real estate, household goods, personal effects, motor vehicles, and insurance may be completely or partially excluded from countable resources depending on their value and the applicant's circumstances.

Noncountable Assets. Of particular importance for Medicaid planning is an understanding of what assets are excluded from the resource calculation (42 U.S.C. §1382b[a]). Provided that the equity in your principal residence does not exceed $500,000, it is excluded from countable resources if you live there or intend to return home after institutional care or if your spouse or other qualified family member lives there (42 U.S.C. §1396p[f][1][A]).[5] If the house is sold, the proceeds are exempt if used to purchase another house within three months.

Household goods and personal effects are excluded, as well as one car of any value provided it is used to transport you or a member of your household. Other cars are considered countable resources. If you have property used in a trade or business that is essential for self-support, such property is not counted.

Your life insurance is excludable to the extent that the combined face value does not exceed $1,500. If the value exceeds $1,500, all cash surrender value is a countable resource. Burial spaces for yourself or your immediate family are also exempt. Likewise, prepaid burial expenses or a burial fund up to a value of $1,500 for an individual and $3,000 for a couple is excluded.

Resource Spend-Down. If your countable resources exceed the limit, you may still be able to qualify for Medicaid by spending down those resources on your medical care. For example, Jean enters a nursing home when she has savings of $20,000. After she spends $18,000 for the cost of her nursing home care, she will have only $2,000 and will meet the resource eligibility requirement. Individuals may also spend down by converting a countable resource into an exempt asset or by paying for their own support needs or those of their spouse. For example, Rachael and Ralph are married. Ralph has to enter a nursing home. In order to meet the resource eligibility limits, they buy a new car for Rachael. Because it is the only car they own, it is an excludable resource.

Income

The income limits for Medicaid applicants depend on the size of the applicant's household. In 2010 the income standard for a household of one was $674 per month and $1,011 for a household of two. For applicants seeking home and community-based waiver services, the income limit is usually more generous. There are also special rules for married couples when one spouse plans to reside in a nursing home and the other will remain in the community. These rules, known as the spousal impoverishment protections, are discussed in the next section.

If an applicant's income exceeds the income limit, the applicant can deduct incurred medical expenses to achieve eligibility. For example, Tina, age 68, lives in an apartment and has a monthly countable income of $800. Tina has medical bills of $150 a month. After deducting the $150, Tina has countable income of $650 and so is eligible for Medicaid.

In determining income eligibility for medically needy individuals who reside in nursing homes, states have a choice between two methods—the spend-down method or the income-cap method. The spend-down method requires the applicant to spend all of his or her income on medical care except for a personal needs allowance. The monthly amount of the personal needs allowance varies by state, but a single individual may keep at least $30 and a married couple may keep at least $60. Provided the applicant also meets the resource test, Medicaid will pay the portion of the nursing home expenses not covered by the applicant's income.

Consider the example of Janet, who resides in a nursing home and has no resources. Her income is $2,030 per month, which exceeds the $674 income limit to qualify her as categorically needy under Medicaid. Because her nursing home monthly cost is $5,500, Janet qualifies as medically needy. Janet can retain $30 as a personal needs allowance, but she must apply the remaining $2,000 to her monthly nursing home bill. Medicaid will pay the additional cost of her nursing home care.

Income-cap states have a more restrictive income standard for eligibility. These states set a fixed cap on an applicant's monthly income—usually at 300 percent of the SSI income benefit. In 2010, this cap in most states was $2,022 (3 x $674). An applicant whose income exceeds this limit by even $1 is not eligible for Medicaid. The income-cap states are Alabama, Alaska, Colorado, Connecticut (uses income cap only for those receiving home health care services), Delaware, Idaho, Mississippi, Nevada, New Mexico, Oregon, South Carolina, South Dakota, and Wyoming. Several other states—Arizona, Arkansas, Florida, Iowa, Louisiana, and Oklahoma—do not permit the cost of nursing home expenses to be used to spend down excess income and so as a practical matter are income-cap states. Texas is also an income-cap state with respect to seniors because it excludes the aged from its spend-down, medically needy program.

In income-cap states, you can still obtain Medicaid eligibility by assigning your excess income to what is known as a Miller trust (42 U.S.C. §1396p[d]). Under a Miller trust, a trustee collects and holds all of your income and has authority to distribute monthly income to you only up to the income-cap amount. At your death, the state has a claim on the trust assets for all amounts paid by Medicaid on your behalf.

Special Considerations for Married Individuals

When a married individual enters a nursing home (the institutionalized spouse), the costs of his or her care can place a significant financial strain on the other spouse (the community spouse). Medicaid rules for a married, institutionalized applicant are designed to help the community spouse have adequate income and resources. The rules allow a married individual to become medically eligible for Medicaid without requiring the noninstitutionalized spouse to become destitute. The noninstitutionalized spouse is known as the "community spouse" regardless of where he or she lives so long as it is not in a nursing home.

Only the income of the institutionalized spouse is counted in determining eligibility for Medicaid (42 U.S.C. §1396r-5[b][1]). None of the income of the community spouse is counted. This is known as the "name on the check rule" because it is the name on the check that determines whether the income is considered to be that of the institutionalized or the community spouse. If the institutionalized spouse and the community spouse receive joint income, such as interest payments from jointly held investments, each is considered to be the owner of one-half of the income (42 U.S.C. §1396r-5[b][2][A] and [C]).The community spouse does not have to spend any of his or her income on the cost of the nursing home for the institutionalized spouse.

If the couple lives in an income-cap state and the institutionalized spouse has income that exceeds the income limit, it may be possible to go to court for an order of separate maintenance. Under this order, the institutionalized spouse signs a qualified domestic relations order that assigns part of his or her pension income to the community spouse and thereby reduces the income of the institutionalized spouse to an amount that is below the income cap.

Resources

Whereas the income test considers only the income of the institutionalized spouse, the resource test considers all resources of the married couple (42 U.S.C. §1396r-5[c]). All countable resources owned by the couple, regardless of how owned or titled, are considered available resources that must be spent down before either spouse is eligible for Medicaid. The resources are valued as of the first day of the month of continuous nursing home residency that is expected to last thirty days (42 U.S.C. §1396r-5[c][1][A]). This determination of value is known as the snapshot; it has important consequences for the community spouse.

On the snapshot date, only countable resources are considered, and each is valued at its fair market value. What qualifies as a countable resource is determined by the SSI rules. Once the couple's countable resources have been established, the amount of those resources that may be retained by the community spouse can be determined. Resources that cannot be retained by the community spouse must be spent down until the institutionalized spouse meets the eligibility requirement.

Community Spouse Resource and Income Rights

Community Spouse Resource Allowance. To avoid reducing the community spouse to poverty while the institutionalized spouse spends down income and assets, Medicaid allows the community spouse to retain all of his or her income and some resources, known as the Community Spouse Resource Allowance (42 U.S.C. §1396r-5[f]). The amount of the retained resources is adjusted annually for inflation. In 2010, federal law permitted states to award the community spouse a resource allowance between $21,912 and $109,560. A few states grant the community spouse the lesser of the maximum amount ($109,560) or all of the couple's countable resources. Most states, however, grant the community spouse one-half of the countable resources, up to the maximum amount of $109,560.

Consider the following examples. If a couple had $120,000 of countable resources in 2010, some states would permit the community spouse to retain the maximum of $109,560, but most states would permit a resource allowance of only $60,000 (half of the countable resources). If the couple had $250,000 in countable resources, the community spouse could retain $109,560. If the couple had only $25,000 in countable resources, the community spouse could retain the minimum of $21,912 and, in a few states, $25,000. If the couple had only $10,000 in countable assets, the community spouse would keep all $10,000 in all states.

Minimum Monthly Maintenance Needs Allowance. In addition to the Community Spouse Resource Allowance, the community spouse is permitted to have a minimum income. If his or her own income is below that allowed amount, known as the Minimum Monthly Maintenance Needs Allowance (MMMNA), the community spouse can claim income from the institutionalized spouse (42 U.S.C. §1396r-5[d]). The MMMNA is equal to 150 percent of the federal poverty level for a two-person household ($1,821.25 as of July 1, 2009) plus an excess shelter allowance that together cannot exceed the annual cap of $2,739 per month in 2010 (adjusted annually).[6] The excess shelter allowance is the sum of the spouse's expenses for rent or mortgage payments, taxes, insurance, condominium or cooperative maintenance charges, and either a standard utility allowance or the spouse's actual utility expense. If that sum exceeds 30 percent of the MMMNA, the community spouse may be permitted to keep an increased allowance up to the annual cap.

For example, Lucy, the community spouse, has a monthly income of $1,000. She is permitted to claim at least $821.25 of monthly income from her institutionalized spouse. If she could demonstrate excess shelter costs, she could further increase her MMMNA up to a maximum in 2010 of $2,739. A few states have adopted the maximum dollar amount as the MMMNA for every community spouse.

If the institutionalized spouse is under a court order to provide support to the community spouse, the income must be diverted from the institutionalized spouse to the community spouse even if the amount exceeds the MMMNA. Therefore, a community spouse who is dissatisfied with the amount of the MMMNA can seek more support by suing the institutionalized spouse. The community spouse may also request a hearing from a state Medicaid agency if not satisfied with the MMMNA and can ask for additional income based on exceptional circumstances such as costly medical expenses.

Income First Rules. If the community spouse's income is below the MMMNA amount, states must allow the community spouse to keep that portion of the institutionalized spouse's income necessary to bring the community spouse's monthly income up to the MMMNA amount (42 U.S.C.

§1396r-5[d]). For example, George, the community spouse, has a monthly income of $1,500 and is entitled to an MMMNA of $2,000. He is entitled to $500 a month from the income of his institutionalized spouse. If his institutionalized spouse's income is less than the amount needed to meet the MMMNA, for example, the institutionalized spouse has only $400 a month income, George will be given all of his spouse's income minus the $30 personal needs allowance, or $370. George, however, is still short $130. The shortfall will be made up by an increase in George's Community Spouse Resource Allowance. He will be allowed to keep additional resources equal to an amount that if invested or used to purchase an annuity would create the necessary additional income of $130.

Planning Techniques for Married Couples

Married couples will want to consider methods of creating eligibility for Medicaid while preserving assets for use by the community spouse. The following are some of the planning techniques to help couples retain income and resources.

Repayment of Debts by Institutionalized Spouse. The snapshot calculation of a couple's total, countable resources is made on the first day of entry into a nursing home. After the calculation of the community spouse's resource allowance has been made, the institutionalized spouse must spend down the remaining resources before becoming eligible for Medicaid. Fortunately, there is no requirement that the institutionalized spouse spend his or her allocation solely on medical care. Institutionalized spouses may spend down their resources on items that will benefit the community spouse. For example, any outstanding debts of the couple should be paid for by the institutionalized spouse. This could include a mortgage, car loan, and credit card debt. Couples can even accumulate debt before the entry into a nursing home with the intent that it will be paid off by the institutionalized spouse.

Conversion of Countable Resources into Exempt Assets. If the couple owns their residence, a number of techniques to preserve assets for the community spouse exist. After the snapshot, the institutionalized spouse should pay all real estate taxes. By paying the taxes, the institutionalized spouse is spending down countable resources while simultaneously benefiting the community spouse and preserving the community spouse's portion of the assets. The institutionalized spouse can purchase a reasonable amount of household goods and pay for any repairs or improvements to the home. Because the value of one car is an excluded asset, the institutionalized spouse may want to purchase a new car for the community spouse soon after the day of the snapshot. A couple can even purchase a new home as a means of spending down the resources of the institutionalized spouse.

Changing Beneficiaries. Many couples have life insurance that names the partner as the beneficiary. A community spouse who owns life insurance should remove the institutionalized spouse as the beneficiary in order to protect the death benefit in the event that the community spouse dies first. The name of the institutionalized spouse should be removed because any funds paid to him or her would be spent on nursing home care. For the same reason, no bank accounts of the community spouse should name the institutionalized spouse as a beneficiary, and the will of the community spouse should leave only the statutorily required minimum to the institutionalized spouse.

Asset Transfers

Look-Back Period and Period of Ineligibility

Many older Americans would like to create Medicaid eligibility by giving away assets to their family members rather than spending them down on their own care. Unfortunately, gifts by Medicaid applicants or their spouses may trigger a period of ineligibility for Medicaid benefits (42 U.S.C. §1396p). The Medicaid application for nursing home benefits requires that the applicant disclose any gifts made within sixty months prior to the application. For gifts made before February 8, 2006, the disclosure period is thirty-six months. These sixty (or thirty-six) months are known as the look-back period, and all assets transferred for less than fair market value during this period must be reported on the Medicaid application.

If an applicant made a gift during the look-back period, the length of Medicaid ineligibility will depend on the gift's value. The period of ineligibility is determined by dividing the gift's value by the average monthly cost of nursing home care in the applicant's state. The result (rounded up if not a whole number) is the number of months of Medicaid ineligibility. For example, if Tom gives $40,000 to his daughter, and the state average monthly cost of nursing home care is $5,000, he will be ineligible for Medicaid for eight months.

The period of ineligibility begins the month the individual is in a nursing home or is medically eligible for nursing home care and, except for the penalty period, would "otherwise" be eligible for Medicaid. For example, on June 1, 2007, Ben gives away $50,000 to his son. The average monthly nursing home cost in Ben's state is $5,000. On June 1, 2009, two years after he made the gift, Ben moves into a nursing home with $4,000 of countable resources and a monthly income of $2,500. The nursing home charges $6,500 per month. By July 1, 2009, Ben has exhausted his savings and his income is less than his monthly cost of care. Ben's state is an income spend-down state, and so he is now "otherwise" eligible for Medicaid. His gift on June 1, 2007, within the sixty-month look-back period, causes ten months of ineligibility, which begins to run on July 1, 2009, the date when he is otherwise eligible for Medicaid. As a result of the penalty period, Ben will not be eligible for Medicaid until May 1, 2010.

If an individual gives away assets but does not apply for Medicaid until after the look-back period, the gift will not affect eligibility. When the individual eventually submits an application, the gift does not have to be revealed on the Medicaid application. If a couple have made gifts and both later apply for Medicaid nursing benefits, the state must apportion the period of ineligibility between them. The state may not create a single period of ineligibility and apply it to both individuals.

Provided an individual can show that assets were transferred for a reason other than to qualify for Medicaid, no period of ineligibility will accrue. However, this argument is rarely successful. The applicant must provide convincing evidence about the specific purpose for which the assets were transferred in order to qualify for the exception. States can grant hardship waivers that permit eligibility even though the applicant made disqualifying transfers, but states are very reluctant to grant such waivers.

Depending on the state, community spouses may or may not be permitted to give away resources. Some states allow the community spouse to give away assets after the institutionalized spouse has become eligible; others maintain that any gifts by the community spouse after eligibility trigger a period of ineligibility for the institutionalized spouse.

Exempt Gifts
Some gifts do not trigger a period of ineligibility. These include gifts to the applicant's spouse or to another for the sole benefit of the applicant's spouse. Also included are gifts to a blind or disabled child of the applicant or to a trust solely for the benefit of that child.

Transfer of Home
The home is an exempt resource if the equity value does not exceed $500,000 (or up to $750,000 if the state so elects) and the community spouse is living in it at the time available resources are calculated. In the case of a single individual, the home is also an exempt resource as long as the individual expects to return to it (even if that expectation is unreasonable). A few states deem the home a countable resource for a single individual after a set period of time, such as a year.

Though the home is normally exempt, gifts of a home will typically trigger a period of ineligibility, because the home will lose its exempt status once transferred. However, certain transfers will not trigger a penalty period. If the house is given to a spouse, a child under the age of 21, or a child who is blind or permanently and totally disabled, the gift will not cause a period of ineligibility for the applicant. Furthermore, if the house is given to the applicant's sibling who has an equity interest in the home and who resided in it for at least a year prior to the application, the gift will not cause ineligibility. Neither will a penalty period be triggered if the house is given to a child who resided in it for at least two years immediately before the applicant was institutionalized and who provided care that permitted the applicant to reside at home.

The state may forgo the penalty period if it determines that denying eligibility would be an undue hardship on the applicant. Undue hardship is interpreted as meaning that the transfer penalty would endanger the applicant's life by depriving him or her of medical care.

If the house is titled in the name of the institutionalized spouse or is jointly owned, the standard practice is to retitle the house in the name of the community spouse. Retitling the house protects its value in the event that the community spouse predeceases the institutionalized spouse. If the house were left to the institutionalized spouse, it would likely become an available resource and as such would disqualify the institutionalized spouse for Medicaid. In many states, after the institutionalized spouse has become eligible for Medicaid, the community spouse may transfer the home to a third party, such as a child, without affecting the institutionalized spouse's eligibility.

Gifts in Trust

Revocable trusts do not shield assets from counting as available resources to the Medicaid applicant (42 U.S.C. §1396p[d]). Because the creator of the revocable trust can revoke it and reclaim the trust assets, all the trust income and assets are considered available resources. The effects of an irrevocable trust are more complicated. If the applicant or the applicant's spouse transfers assets to an irrevocable trust that cannot distribute principal for the benefit of the applicant or spouse (i.e., the trust can make distributions only to a third party), the assets may trigger a penalty period. The look-back period for trusts is sixty months. If the trust can make distributions to the applicant or to his or her spouse, the trust is considered an available resource for the applicant. If a trust makes distributions of principal or income to a third party, the distributions are considered gifts.

Estate Recovery

The federal Medicaid statute requires states to attempt recovery of Medicaid payments from the estates of those who were provided benefits (42 U.S.C. §1396p[b][1][B]). The state has the right to recover from the beneficiary's estate or to enforce a Medicaid lien when the Medicaid beneficiary's property is sold. The beneficiary's estate is all real and personal property included in the state's definition of a probate estate. The state may also include other assets in which the beneficiary had a legal interest, such as jointly titled assets or assets in trust.

A lien on the house cannot be enforced so long as the house is occupied by certain individuals. For example, a lien cannot be enforced while a surviving spouse or a minor, blind, or disabled child is living in the house. The same is true while a sibling is living there, provided the sibling has an equity interest in the house and resided there for at least one year prior to the beneficiary's institutionalization. If the house sharer is a child who is not a minor or is not blind or disabled, the child must have resided in the house for at least two years prior to institutionalization and must prove that he or she provided care to the Medicaid beneficiary that permitted the beneficiary to live at home. A state may waive recovery if it would cause an undue hardship, such as where the property is the sole source of income for survivors. A few states have ignored the rule and do not enforce estate recovery.

Long-Term Care Insurance

Seniors who wish to pass on their assets or avoid burdening their children often purchase long-term care insurance. Long-term care insurance policies are sold by private insurance companies, not by the federal government. The policies guarantee a fixed monthly cash payment in the event the insured individual enters a nursing home or assisted living facility or requires long-term care at home.

Reasons to Purchase Long-Term Care Insurance

Three reasons exist for purchasing long-term care insurance. First, you may want to protect the value of your estate against the potentially high costs of long-term care. Second, you may want to protect your spouse or yourself against a lower standard of living if one of you needs nursing home care. And third, you may fear relying on Medicaid.

If your concern is maintaining the size of your estate, you should consider whether preservation of the estate is worth the cost of paying long-term care insurance premiums for potentially twenty or thirty years. You should consider how much you would be willing to spend from your estate on long-term care and then purchase only enough insurance to cover the additional risk. For example, Alison and Art, both age 66, own a house worth $250,000 and have savings of $300,000. Each has income from a pension and Social Security of $40,000 a year, for a total income of $80,000. They buy long-term care insurance that will pay $200 a day for up to three years for each of them. In other words, the maximum benefits from the policy are approximately $219,000 per person or $438,000 for both. They buy the policy because they are willing to spend some of their income and resources on their long-term care but do not want to exhaust all of their savings on their care. They have three children and four grandchildren and hope to pass some money to them when they die.

One alternative to long-term care insurance is life insurance if your concern is depletion of your estate. Life insurance is typically less expensive, particularly second-to-die policies that do not pay death benefits until the last of the two spouses dies. Although life insurance will not help pay for long-term care needs, it can be viewed as replacement money for the money spent on long-term care. If the estate is depleted because of nursing home expenses, the life insurance will ensure the heirs an estate of a meaningful size.

If your concern is protecting the quality of your life or that of your spouse in the event one of you needs expensive nursing home care, you should consider whether you would likely qualify for Medicaid under the spousal impoverishment protections and calculate what the community spouse would be able to retain under those rules versus the cost of maintaining long-term care insurance. Even though Medicaid does allow the community spouse to retain some assets and income, long-term care insurance can reduce the risk of having to divest assets to that level.

For example, Caitlin and Curtis buy a policy with a ninety-day elimination period that pays $200 a day for five years. Curtis develops dementia. As the disease progresses, he moves to an assisted living facility at a cost of $150 a day. After ninety days, the couple has spent $13,500 on his care, which they paid from their savings. Curtis's condition has worsened, and so he moves to a nursing home that costs $250 a day. Their long-term care policy begins to pay $200 a day. After three years in the nursing home, Curtis dies. The nursing home cost to the couple was $50 a day for three years or $54,750. In total, the couple's cost of care for Curtis in assisted living and in the nursing home was $68,250. Although they had only $250,000 in savings, thanks to the long-term care insurance, the couple was able to meet the cost without resorting to Medicaid and its spend-down requirements.

If you want long-term care insurance because you are reluctant to rely on Medicaid, it is important to look realistically at the trade-offs. If you fear that Medicaid will not be available in the future, that fear is probably unfounded. Public subsidy of long-term care is not going away so long as so many cannot afford the cost of long-term care. And if you would presently qualify for Medicaid, then long-term care insurance is not cost-justified for you.

If you fear that the quality of care in Medicaid-reimbursed nursing homes will decline, there is no doubt that individuals with long-term care insurance who can privately pay for nursing home care will have a greater choice of nursing homes. With that said, more than 90 percent of nursing homes accept Medicare and Medicaid reimbursement, and there is typically no difference in care between residents on Medicaid and those who are paying for their care with private funds and long-term care insurance.

Probably more realistic are concerns that Medicaid waiver services in your home or in the community (such as adult day care) might not be available when you need them because of long waiting lists or the possibility that your assets or income would disqualify you for such services. Long-term care insurance that includes a home care benefit can help alleviate those concerns.

Choosing a Long-Term Care Policy

More than one hundred companies offer long-term care insurance, though many that once sold such policies have retreated from the market because it is so difficult to estimate the cost of future benefit payouts. The most important aspect of choosing a policy is its coverage, including the scope—what it will pay and for what type of care (e.g., nursing home, assisted living facility, in your own home) and the terms under which coverage will begin, including the length of any elimination period before benefits are payable and the triggers for the onset of coverage. You will also want to consider whether the policy is "tax qualified" and whether the policy qualifies as a "partnership policy" under your state's Medicaid law.

Coverage. Because there is no standard long-term care coverage, you should examine each policy carefully. Most policies provide coverage for care in nursing homes, but you should consider whether home care and coverage for an assisted living facility are also important to you. The scope of coverage will impact the cost of the premiums.

Most long-term care insurance policies are pure indemnity, that is, they pay a fixed dollar amount for each day that you are in a nursing home or assisted living facility or are receiving home care. Other policies pay only for the actual daily cost of care up to a fixed amount. Some policies also have an inflation-adjustment rider that will increase the daily benefit by a set percentage, typically 5 percent per year. Given the rising cost of long-term care, you should consider purchasing the inflation-adjustment rider to assure that the benefit amount will keep pace with the actual cost of care.

Long-term care insurance generally pays benefits if you are certified by a physician as having cognitive deficits, such as those caused by dementia, or are unable to do two of the five activities of daily living:

- bathing
- toileting
- eating
- dressing
- transferring (getting out of a bed or chair without assistance)

Many policies pay benefits for home care as well as nursing home care. Often home care benefits are one-half as generous as benefits paid if you are in a nursing home or assisted living facility. For example, the policy might pay $150 per day for nursing home care or care in an assisted living facility, but only $75 a day for care received at home. Because nursing home care is usually more than $200 a day, long-term care insurance will generally not meet the entire cost. It may cover most of the cost of care in an assisted living facility.

A long-term care insurance policy may limit how long it will pay benefits. Though it is possible to buy a policy that will pay benefits for the life of the insured, many pay benefits for two, three, or five years. The longer the policy pays benefits, the higher the premiums are. Time limits on benefit payments apply without regard to whether you are at home or in an institution, although some policies have separate time limits for home and institutionalized benefits. For example, Jack owns a long-term care insurance policy that pays home care benefits for two years and institutional care benefits for five. Jack receives eighteen months of home care benefits and then moves into a nursing home. Under the terms of the policy, he will still have five years worth of institutionalized care benefits.

Some policies have an "elimination" period of thirty, sixty, or ninety days, meaning the benefits are not paid until after you first meet the qualifications for receiving benefits for the length of the elimination period. For example, Pauline enters an assisted living facility because she cannot perform two activities of daily living. She qualifies for the daily benefit under her long-term care insurance policy, but the policy has a sixty-day elimination period. She must wait sixty days before she will begin to receive benefits.

Choosing a longer elimination period can reduce your premium costs. Some policies do not require the elimination period to be consecutive days. These policies have an accumulation period during which the total number of elimination days may be met. For example, if a policy has a ninety-day elimination period and a nine-month accumulation period, you will begin receiving benefits as soon as you spend ninety days in a nursing facility, even if they are not consecutive, provided they occur during a nine-month period.

Long-term care policies may exclude coverage for mental illness other than Alzheimer's disease or other forms of dementia. Often policies will not cover treatment for alcoholism, drug addiction, illness related to wartime injuries or sickness, and treatment necessitated by attempted suicide. Preexisting conditions may not be covered or may be excluded from coverage for the first six months that the policy is in effect. You generally must submit to a physical examination to qualify for long-term care insurance. Based on the physical or other factors, many applicants are denied. An estimated 25 to 50 percent of applicants are turned down by at least one insurance company.

Age, at least until age 84, will not exclude an individual from purchasing a policy, as policies are generally sold to individuals between ages 50 and 84. The annual premium rises with the age at which the policy is purchased. Premiums are much lower when the policy is purchased at age 60 than at age 75. Plus the likelihood of being denied insurance increases with age. Once you purchase a policy, the premium will not be raised unless the company raises premiums for all similar policies; unfortunately, that is very likely to occur.

Long-term care insurance is costly because you will need to keep the policy in effect for the rest of your life. A 65-year-old buyer, for example, can

expect to pay premiums for twenty to thirty years. Although many purchasers find the annual cost of the insurance to be very burdensome, once
purchased it makes no sense to let a policy lapse because the likelihood of
needing the benefits increases with age.

Almost all long-term care insurance policies are indefinitely renewable
unless the company withdraws coverage from the state in which the insured
resides. The policy can be terminated, however, if the insured does not pay
the premium, but there are usually antilapse protections if the failure to pay
the premium is due to a condition over which the insured has no control,
such as mental incapacity. Most policies will waive the premium when the
insured begins to collect benefits. This provision is usually standard in policies, but you should check the particular policy. If you voluntarily terminate
a policy, generally the coverage is terminated with no credit for prior premiums paid.

Federal Tax Benefits. The benefits paid by a long-term care insurance policy
are not taxable as income if the policy is "tax qualified" (I.R.C. §7702B[a][1]).
Most, but not all, policies are tax qualified, which means that the policy is
guaranteed renewable, does not require prior hospitalization to trigger the
payment of benefits, and complies with the Long-Term Care Insurance
Model Regulation and the Long-Term Care Insurance Model Act developed
by the National Association of Insurance Commissioners (NAIC) (I.R.C.
§7702B[b]). The premiums for such insurance can be deducted as a medical
expense, though the amount that can be deducted is capped and increases with
the age of the taxpayer (I.R.C. §213[d][1][C]). In 2010 a taxpayer age 70 or
older could deduct up to $4,110 in premiums. This amount is adjusted annu-
ally for inflation. Only taxpayers who itemize deductions (rather than claiming the standard deduction) may take this deduction and then only if all medical expenses, including the allowable portion of the long-term care insurance
premium, exceed 7½ percent of adjusted gross income.

Medicaid Long-Term Care Insurance Partnerships. In order to encourage
more private payment of long-term care and less reliance on Medicaid,
Congress enacted legislation promoting state long-term care insurance partnership plans (42 U.S.C. §1396p[b][1][C]). An individual who has received
benefits under a long-term care partnership insurance policy will be permitted to retain assets up to the amount of those benefits. For example, if Joan
owned a long-term care insurance policy that paid her $150,000 in benefits
and she then applied for Medicaid, Joan would be permitted to own
$150,000 in countable resources and still be eligible for Medicaid. Of course,
Joan would still have to meet the state income requirements. To be eligible
for partnership policy status, the long-term care insurance policy must meet

the specifications of the Long-Term Care Insurance Model Act and offer in-flation protection by increasing the benefits over the life of the policy. About one-half the states have adopted partnership plans.

Tips for Purchasing Long-Term Care Insurance

The National Association of Insurance Commissioners provides sugges-tions on shopping for and purchasing long-term care insurance. It suggests that you check with several companies and agents and compare premiums against similar benefits. If the company cannot or will not explain the terms of the policy, you should not purchase a policy from the company. You should purchase only one good policy instead of stacking multiple policies. NAIC also urges that you disclose your entire medical history. If you do not disclose everything, the company may be permitted to refuse to pay benefits or even cancel the policy. Although most states require insurance companies to provide purchasers with a thirty-day cancellation period in which they can obtain a full refund, you should always check how much time you have to cancel with full refund rights.

Notes

1. Kaiser Commission on Medicaid and the Uninsured, *Medicaid: An Overview of Spending on "Mandatory" vs. "Optional" Populations and Services*, Issue Paper No. 7331 (Menlo Park, CA: Kaiser Family Foundation, June 2005), 8, available at http://www.kff.org/medicaid/upload/Medicaid-An-Overview-of-Spending-on.pdf.

2. *Id*. at 7.

3. *Id*. at 8.

4. This rule applies to transfers on or after February 8, 2006. Prior to this date, the look-back for asset transfers other than to a trust was thirty-six months and sixty months for transfers to a trust (42 U.S.C. §1396p[c][B][i]).

5. States may elect a higher equity cap not to exceed $750,000 (42 U.S.C. §1396p[f][1][B]).

6. The MMMNA amounts may vary slightly by state.

For More Information

Centers for Medicare and Medicaid Services
(http://www.cms.hhs.gov)

Follow the links for Medicaid to find information about many Medicaid-re-lated topics.

National Association of Insurance Commissioners
(http://www.naic.org)

Follow the consumer links to find educational information tailored to the insurance needs of seniors. Also find complaint and financial information about specific insurance companies.

National SHIP Resource Center
(http://www.shiptalk.org)

Find information about free one-on-one counseling to help you make decisions about your insurance needs, including long-term care insurance.

7

Housing

Did You Know?

- Hiring regular help at home may be less costly than moving to assisted living.
- Medicaid-funded help may be available at home as well as in a nursing home.
- Age-restricted housing may prohibit children not only as residents, but also as overnight guests.
- An owners association may have the right to change the rules after you buy your condominium or house in a planned community.
- An assisted living facility may have the right to terminate your contract even if your heath crisis, such as a stroke, is temporary.
- Nursing Home Compare is a federal website that provides information about the quality of all nursing homes that receive Medicare or Medicaid funding.

Where you live has a significant impact on your overall quality of life. The need to choose a new place to live usually results from a change in circumstances such as marriage, divorce, different employment, children leaving home, retirement, or a health crisis. Physical changes that come with advanced age are also common reasons that seniors move.

If you are a young senior thinking about a move at retirement or when the children leave home, you are likely to want a place that will meet your present interests as well as your future needs. You may want a quiet community that includes easy access to favorite activities such as golf, tennis, fishing, or cultural events. If you are an older senior, you may want housing options that also offer supportive services. These can range from limited assistance, such as light housekeeping, laundry services, and group meals, to more extensive assistance, such as help with dressing and bathing and skilled nursing care.

Just as seniors are a very diverse group in terms of age, health, and needs, so are senior housing options diverse in terms of services offered, eligibility requirements, and cost. Often the housing options that are most widely promoted are those that produce income for someone else—the developers of retirement communities or the service providers associated with assisted living facilities. This is why retirement communities and assisted living facilities are so aggressively marketed to seniors.

Equally adequate, or perhaps even better, options may exist for "aging in place" in your own house, condominium, or apartment. Information about these options, however, may be more difficult to find. The senior who wants to age in place may have to spend more effort to locate and coordinate needed services than would be required if he or she moved to a retirement community or assisted living facility. There is almost always a cost and convenience trade-off when choosing among senior housing options.

The remainder of this chapter provides an overview of senior housing options as well as important factors to be considered with each. First, the option of aging in place is explored, followed by a discussion of special age-restricted housing alternatives. Next, different types of independent living retirement housing are described, followed by an examination of supportive housing options that offer some degree of assistive services. Finally, residence in a nursing home is discussed for seniors with greater care and medical needs.

Aging in Place

For many seniors, the best housing is the house, condominium, or apartment where they presently live. Memories, friends, and familiar neighborhood places are some of the reasons that seniors want to age in place. Even though you may want to stay connected to the home, people, and places that are familiar, you may also fear what will happen if your health or that of your spouse deteriorates. The main challenge of aging in place is how to get help if your needs become greater than your ability to meet them.

Although aging in place presents challenges, the advantages go beyond the mere comfort of staying in a familiar situation. A move to a new residence has real downsides. It not only costs money to move; it also takes a great deal of physical and psychological energy. Preparing one residence for sale while finding a new place to live can be very stressful.

Yet aging in place also has disadvantages. You may have too much money tied up in a house that is too big and expensive to maintain. As you age, so does your house, and you may be less capable of maintaining it. What were routine tasks in the past may now require hired help to accomplish. Regular chores, such as cutting the lawn, raking leaves, cleaning gutters, and even taking out the garbage, may become difficult or impossible because of chronic health conditions or loss of stamina.

Sometimes changes take place in a neighborhood or community that make it less safe or appropriate for senior living. If you live in a city, essential services may have relocated from a central to a suburban location. If you live in the suburbs, necessary services may be accessible only if you can drive. The following discussion examines other important factors to consider if you want to age in place.

Practical Responses

Seniors who want to age in place can do so, but it takes planning. You must determine how to adapt your home to the realities of old age and do so with little or no assistance from the government. Unfortunately, there is little public money or support available for seniors trying to age in place. However, private solutions are available for seniors who are flexible and imaginative.

Paying the Bills. You must first calculate current monthly housing expenses. This calculation should include converting annual expenses (such as property taxes and insurance) and extraordinary expenses (such as periodic roof repair) into estimated monthly amounts. If you have enough income to meet those expenses (as well as the other costs of living), the next step is to consider what improvements would make your home more "senior friendly."

Examples of senior-friendly improvements include the installation of grab bars in the bathroom or the addition of a bathroom on the first floor. Moving a washer and dryer from the basement to the first floor is another. Some seniors who have difficulty climbing stairs convert an underused first floor dining room into their bedroom. Of course, using capital to modify the house should only be done if you can afford to spend part of your savings. When the house is eventually sold, the improvements may not increase the value of the home because many younger purchasers will either not care about the modifications or may even have to pay to reverse them, such as reconverting the bedroom into a dining room.

House Sharing with a Relative. If you cannot afford the cost of aging in place, there are alternatives. One is to invite someone to share the house. Many seniors ask a relative, typically an adult child or grandchild, to live with them. Some only ask the relative to share expenses, whereas others ask for at least some rent. Local zoning laws probably do not prohibit house sharing as long as no rent is paid because zoning laws do not prohibit two unmarried or even unrelated persons from living together.

House sharing can benefit both participants, but problems can arise, even when the house sharer is a relative. You should clearly define what you expect from the relationship. For example, in return for not requiring rent, do you expect the house sharer to take care of upkeep and minor repairs? Or do you expect the house sharer to provide your transportation to doctor's appointments, church, and the grocery store? Are you going to share meals, and, if so, who pays for the groceries, who cooks, and who cleans up? Seemingly minor points such as these, if not clearly answered, can lead to friction and possibly end the arrangement. It is far better to discuss possible problem areas upfront.

Another potential problem is the possibility that the person sharing your house will take advantage of you if you later become dependent because of declining physical or mental health. Exploitation of older persons takes many forms. It may be financial, such as using your money in ways that do not benefit you, or physical, such as neglecting to provide you with needed food and care. If you choose to participate in a house sharing arrangement and think that you may eventually become dependent on the house sharer, it is a good idea to have another relative or friend visit regularly to monitor your well-being.

Even though dependency on the house sharer may be unavoidable, you should not unnecessarily increase it by choosing the house sharer to serve as your agent under a power of attorney. A power of attorney is a legal document that gives the agent control over your property and finances (see Chapter 9 for general information about a power of attorney). Although appointing the house sharer to handle your financial affairs seems convenient, it creates big risks. If you are already physically dependent on the house sharing relative, that individual has a great deal of control over your person. Giving that same individual control over your property further increases the opportunity for financial exploitation. The solution is either to name someone other than the house sharer as agent under a power of attorney or to name another person as a co-agent with the house sharer to serve as a check-and-balance.

House Sharing with a Stranger. Some seniors are willing to share their house with a stranger. If rent is involved, the local zoning law may prohibit the arrangement. Such laws, however, are rarely enforced unless someone complains. Some homeowners do not charge rent but expect the house sharer to "pay" his or her way by handling certain chores, such as taking out the garbage or shoveling snow and doing basic repairs and maintenance.

Unfortunately, inviting a stranger into your house creates serious risks. Some churches, community service organizations, and senior citizen centers help screen potential house sharers. These organizations act as brokers and match interested older homeowners with trustworthy house sharers. If no organization is willing to do so, the necessary background search must be performed by the homeowner, but this is not very practical. It is difficult for an individual to undertake a background check that includes a search of criminal and civil court records, credit records, and employment records, as well as interviews with the prospective house sharer's past and current neighbors.

If you choose to enter into a house sharing arrangement with a relative or someone else, you should check with your insurance agent to see if your homeowner's insurance covers the new house sharer, both for injury to property and person caused by the house sharer and for injury to the house sharer and his or her property.

Reverse Mortgage. If you want to remain in your own home but would rather not enter into a house sharing arrangement to cover expenses, another option to consider is a reverse mortgage. A reverse mortgage is merely a fancy term for taking out a loan and pledging your house as security. What makes a reverse mortgage different from traditional home loans is that repayment is delayed until a triggering event occurs. Common repayment triggers include the homeowner selling the house, no longer living in it, failing to properly maintain or pay the property taxes on it, or dying. Reverse mortgages are not for everyone, but they can provide needed financial resources to seniors who are "house rich and cash poor."

Seniors should carefully consider the costs associated with a reverse mortgage. These costs are substantial and can include onetime charges, such as origination fees and closing costs, as well as fees that accumulate over the length of the loan, such as loan servicing fees and monthly mortgage insurance premiums. A senior borrower may not fully appreciate how sizable these fees may become because they are usually financed as a part of the total loan rather than paid upfront. When the borrower's house is eventually sold, these fees will be deducted from the sale proceeds along with the sums necessary to repay the loan principal and accrued interest.

Consider the example of Ann, age 75, who owns a home worth $150,000. She decides to borrow $60,000 from a bank in the form of a reverse mortgage because her monthly income is not adequate to cover her living expenses. Under the terms of the reverse mortgage, Ann agrees to pay 6 percent annual interest on the unpaid balance of the loan. She will not have to make any payment of principal and interest until she dies, sells the house, or no longer lives in it. If Ann dies at age 80 and her estate sells the house for $165,000, the estate will owe the bank $80,000 as a repayment of the principal and interest as well as accrued loan fees, which will likely total more than $10,000. The remaining sum of approximately $75,000 will go to her estate. By taking out the reverse mortgage, Ann was able to both stay in her home and meet her living expenses. However, to obtain the use of $60,000, Ann in actuality paid approximately $30,000 in interest and fees.

Not all older individuals who take out a reverse mortgage receive a lump sum. Instead, they may choose to establish a line of credit, such as the right to borrow up to $60,000, which they can take in set dollar amounts each month or on an as-needed basis. For example, Bart, age 80, has a house worth $200,000. He arranges with a bank to borrow $400 a month or $4,800 a year for the next twelve years at a rate of 7 percent annual interest. If Bart actually does borrow $400 a month for twelve years, he will owe $57,600 in principal plus interest of approximately $13,400, or a total debt of $71,000. Bart would then be age 92. Assume that Bart continues to live in his house until age 95, when he moves into a nursing home. That move triggers the repayment obligation on the loan. The debt of $71,000 will have grown by the annual interest of 7 percent per year to an additional $15,000. Bart would owe the bank approximately $86,000 to cover the principal and interest on the loan plus accumulated fees, which could total more than $20,000. If he is able to sell his house for $256,000, the bank would receive approximately $106,000 and Bart would keep $150,000.

Although the most common trigger for repayment of a reverse mortgage is the borrower's death or the sale of the house, declining health and the need for assisted living or nursing home care are also significant repayment events. Given the large origination fees and closing costs often associated with reverse mortgages, seniors should think carefully about whether a triggering event is likely to occur sooner rather than later. The proportionate impact of large onetime fees is less the longer the mortgage repayment is delayed. One way in which repayment can be delayed is by a couple taking out a reverse mortgage that conditions repayment when the last of the borrowers dies or when neither borrower is able to live in the house.

One advantage of reverse mortgages is that they are typically nonrecourse, which means that the borrower is not personally liable for the debt. In other words, the lender can look only to the house sale proceeds for repayment of the loan. For example, Carol, age 77, owned a house worth $120,000 in 1997. She took out a reverse mortgage and by age 88 owed the lending bank $90,000. Due to the onset of dementia, she moved into an assisted living facility. In 2008, when her house was sold, the value had fallen to $85,000, so the sale proceeds were insufficient to pay off the entire $90,000 debt. Because the reverse mortgage was nonrecourse, Carol does not owe the bank the $5,000.

Lenders limit the amount of home equity that can be borrowed under a reverse mortgage in order to ensure that there will be sufficient sale proceeds to cover the loan when a triggering event occurs. For example, a lender might limit the amount of a reverse mortgage to no more than 70 percent of the estimated fair market value of the house. The amount of the loan or the limit on the line of credit is also affected by the age of the borrower. The younger the borrower is, the less the lender will loan. Because the loan will not be repaid until the house is sold or the borrower dies (or one of the other triggering events occurs), interest on the debt continues to rise. The lender wants the assurance that the total debt owed—principal, interest, and fees—will not exceed the value of the house when it is finally sold. The younger the borrower is, the greater is the amount of interest that is likely to accrue.

To qualify for a reverse mortgage, a homeowner must usually own the house free and clear of any mortgages or liens. In order to postpone repayment until death or the sale of the house, the homeowner will need to take out an insured reverse mortgage. The Federal Housing Administration (FHA) insures reverse mortgages, as do private lenders.[1] An FHA-insured loan is usually less expensive because it has lower upfront fees and may carry a lower rate of interest. However, an FHA-insured loan is available only if the borrower is at least age 62 (24 C.F.R. §206.33), the borrower holds title to the property (24 C.F.R. §206.35), and the house (or condominium) is his or her principal residence (24 C.F.R. §206.39).

The lender must explain to the borrower how a reverse mortgage works and must also provide the names of third parties who can counsel the borrower about the financial realities and consequences of the loan (24 C.F.R. §206.41). Counseling is mandatory and can cost up to $125 for the hour it typically takes. The lender must also disclose to the borrower all costs of obtaining the mortgage and which charges are not required to obtain the mortgage (24 C.F.R. §206.43). The allowable charges and fees are listed in the federal regulations (24 C.F.R. §206.31). The Housing and Economic Recovery Act of 2008 (Pub. L. No. 110-289) limits fees to a maximum of 2 percent on the first $200,000 borrowed and 1 percent of the balance, subject to a cap of $6,000 (Pub. L. No. 110-289, §2122). The law also prevents lenders from requiring borrowers to purchase additional insurance products, such as an annuity, as a precondition for getting a reverse mortgage.

The amount that can be obtained in the form of an insured reverse mortgage loan is a factor of the borrower's age, the interest rate, and the value of the house. There are limits on the loan amounts that can be insured, but the amounts vary throughout the nation and change over time. You can learn the estimated dollar limits for an insured reverse mortgage in your area by using the reverse mortgage calculator available on the AARP website.[2] Remember, even though a reverse mortgage may provide you with cash to cover living expenses so that you can remain in your home, it is not right for everyone. Before committing to a reverse mortgage, think carefully about all of the costs, the events that could trigger your repayment obligation, and your other options and future needs.

Medicare- and Medicaid-Financed Home Health Care

For some, aging in place requires onsite health care assistance. Medicare provides part-time and intermittent home health care for homebound seniors who need skilled nursing care, home health aides, or physical, speech, or occupational therapy (see Chapter 5 for general information about Medicare eligibility). Medicare home health care, however, is not designed to provide long-term care for a chronic condition. Although Medicare home health care can help you return home after hospitalization or remain home while recovering from a medical incident, such as a stroke, it is not a solution if you need long-term care.

Medicaid, the primary public payer of long-term care in nursing homes, has established a "waiver" program by which states can obtain a federal waiver of the Medicaid requirement that it only reimburse institutionalized care (see Chapter 6 for general information about Medicaid eligibility). A waiver permits the state to apply federal Medicaid dollars to pay for long-term care services delivered in your home. The number of waivers and the type and extent of home health care vary from state to state, as do financial eligibility requirements, such as resource and income limits.

Medicaid waiver care is often combined with other home care assistance programs operated by the state or county or by the local Area Agency on Aging. Every state has Area Agencies on Aging, often called by other names, which operate with federal and state funding to coordinate services for seniors. For example, the state Medicaid waiver program might provide a home health aide for twenty hours a week, which might be supplemented by county-provided homemaker services, Meals-on-Wheels meals, and a visiting nurse. The nature and extent of other home assistance vary considerably depending on the policy of the state and the availability of the services. The regional Area Agencies on Aging can provide information to you about home assistance programs available in your area.

The goal of the waiver program, known in some states as Home and Community-Based Services, is to permit you to live in your own home or community for as long as possible at a cost less than that of living in a nursing home. Some waivers provide help to seniors in residential situations other than a private home. Examples include board and care homes, where the waivers make possible the receipt of medical care that the facility is otherwise not licensed to provide, and domiciliary care homes, usually defined under state law as a home for two to four residents where the homeowner is the caregiver.

Another option for seniors who want to age in place but who need both skilled health care and long-term care is known as the Program of All-Inclusive Care for the Elderly (PACE). PACE relies on an interdisciplinary team and often uses adult day care supplemented by in-home care. Individuals age 55 or older may be eligible for PACE if they need nursing home care but would be able to live in the community if provided with the right help. They must meet state Medicaid income and resource eligibility requirements and must sign an agreement to accept PACE as the sole provider of services. The individual's care needs are reviewed twice a year, and eligibility for PACE is reviewed annually. Participants who are dissatisfied with the quality or level of care may submit a formal grievance as described in the program's grievance procedures.

Adult Day Care

Adult day care provides daily care for seniors who either should not or prefer not to be alone during the day. It is often the critical service that makes aging in place possible for an older adult who can no longer manage all alone. Such individuals usually have a family-member caregiver available in the evening, but adult day care makes it possible for that caregiver to go to work or take care of other responsibilities during the day.

Located throughout the community, adult day care centers are usually open from early in the morning until late afternoon five days a week to accommodate those with whom the older adult lives. A few centers are open on the weekends to provide respite care for families who care for the older adult during the week but seek relief on the weekend.

All adult day care centers feature supervised care, meals, and, usually, exercise classes, music, crafts and, sometimes, field trips. Participants typically arrive in the morning and stay all day. For example, an adult child will leave the older adult at the center in the morning and pick her up at the end of the workday. Some centers provide door-to-door transportation, whereas a few communities provide free or subsidized transportation to and from adult day care centers.

The typical client of an adult day care center is an older senior, usually age 80 or older, frail, and possibly suffering a mild loss of mental capacity. Those who attend adult day care cannot be in need of supervised medical care because adult day care centers are not licensed to provide such care. Many who attend, however, do have some degree of dementia.

Adult day care charges by the day, and the daily cost varies greatly based upon labor costs, but it is usually only 25 to 35 percent of the cost of a nursing home. The centers are often operated by nonprofit institutions, but many of the more than three thousand centers are for-profit businesses. Some Area Agencies on Aging offer subsidized adult day care, and some states have programs that offer assistance to low-income individuals in adult day care. Most long-term care insurance will pay benefits for an individual in adult day care if that individual otherwise meets the criteria for the receipt of benefits.

Age-Restricted Housing

Many seniors prefer to live with other older residents in housing that is open only to persons of a minimum age. Such housing includes apartment houses, condominiums, mobile home parks, subdivisions, villages, and even entire towns. Age-restricted housing is not necessarily designed to meet long-term care needs, but it does promise a safe and secure environment that caters to the needs and interests of older persons.

Age-restricted senior housing often provides special recreational, social, or community activities. The larger communities feature clubs, political activities, educational opportunities, charitable and religious activities, and recreational facilities designed for older residents. For many, just living with other seniors is attractive enough to make age-restricted housing a desirable choice.

Critics complain that it is unnatural to remove seniors from the community, and indeed age-restricted housing does not appeal to all older persons. Nevertheless, age-restricted housing is popular enough that it is exempt from the federal fair housing statute that otherwise bars discrimination based on "familial status" (e.g., no discrimination against families with children under age 18) (42 U.S.C. §3607[b][2]). State fair housing laws and even local ordinances also commonly permit housing that accepts only older residents.

Housing for Older Persons Defined

The federal fair housing law defines housing for older persons as housing that is limited to residents age 55 or older and has at least 80 percent of its units occupied by at least one person age 55 or older (42 U.S.C. §3607[b][2][C]). The alternative is to require all units to be occupied by residents age 62 or older (42 U.S.C. §3607[b][2][B]). The requirement that all residents are age 62 or older is a fixed rule that allows no exceptions. For example, a couple is disqualified if only one is age 62 or older. Imagine that Andy and Ann, when both are age 63, move into a retirement village restricted to those age 62 or older. Ann dies at age 64. A year later, Andy, now age 65, marries Katy, age 60. She will not be permitted to move into the retirement village because she is too young.

The age 55 or older test is more flexible. For example, at age 70, Ben and Betty move into an apartment complex that insists that at least 80 percent of the residents be age 55 or older. Ben dies at age 75. Betty, age 75, and in need of daily assistance, wants her 50-year-old daughter, Dora, to move in with her. The apartment complex permits Dora to move in because at the time 90 percent of the occupants are age 55 or older.

You may notice a number of formalities associated with age-restricted housing. Under the law, such communities must demonstrate an intent to meet the requirement that 80 percent of the residents are at least age 55 or older by publishing and following policies that

- describe the housing as age restricted,
- use advertising directed at those age 55 and older,
- use procedures to verify residents' ages, and
- have and enforce written rules, regulations, and lease provisions that ensure compliance with the law (24 C.F.R. §100.306).

The owner or manager of the facility is responsible for enforcing the age limitations.

Many states have laws that are similar to the federal exception for age-restricted senior housing. California, for example, has the Mobile Home Residency Law, which exempts mobile home parks from the state's general law against age discrimination. In California, mobile home parks may discriminate against those under age 55.

Sometimes underage would-be buyers or renters sue age-restricted housing facilities alleging that they violate the federal Fair Housing Act. Such claims may also be brought by a unit owner in the facility who wants to sell to an underage buyer. Despite exceptions under the act for age-restricted housing, a claim may be successful if the facility has failed to consistently enforce the age restrictions (*Massaro v. Mainlands Section 1 & 2 Civic Ass'n, Inc.*, 3 F.3d 1472 [11th Cir. 1993]).

Types of Age-Restricted Housing

When choosing age-restricted housing, you should consider which type is likely to be most appropriate as you age and perhaps require supportive services. Most age-restricted condominium or apartment houses are not likely to provide much in-unit help. If your ability to care for yourself declines, you may have to move to housing that provides in-unit assistance. For many seniors, the better choice is a retirement community or age-restricted subdivision or planned development. Such communities are more likely to offer supportive services as an option.

There are many self-contained small cities or towns designed exclusively for older residents. They include, for example, Leisure World in Southern California, with more than twenty thousand residents, and Sun City in Arizona, with more than forty-five thousand residents; both feature detached single-family houses and townhouses. Large retirement communities typically have extensive recreational facilities, including golf courses, tennis courts, swimming pools, shuffleboard courts, game rooms, libraries, and studios for arts and crafts, woodworking, and other leisure activities. Residents of these communities can find clubs that cater to almost every interest. To attract less financially secure elderly, some retirement towns feature less expensive manufactured housing or mobile homes.

Although individuals with chronic ailments may find it difficult to take advantage of many of the social or recreational attractions of these communities, other conveniences may still make residence in a retirement community worthwhile. Services such as stores, banks, restaurants, and religious facilities may be close enough to your residence to permit easy access on foot or with the use of a golf cart or personal scooter.

Smaller age-segregated villages typically are not self-contained. Residents must be able to drive to obtain services outside the residential area. If you require supportive assistance, such a community may not be a wise choice. Smaller, gated communities are even more isolated and require the resident to be able to drive out of the community to obtain almost any service. They offer few advantages over nonage-restricted housing for those older persons who need supportive assistance.

Age-restricted housing that only requires 80 percent or more of the units to have at least one resident age 55 or older promises a much greater mix of ages, but the facility may be less aimed at the interests of seniors. For example, it may include some recreational facilities that in general do not appeal to or benefit seniors. Also keep in mind that a facility that meets the age 55 and older exemption to the federal Fair Housing Act may legally exclude children, but not all do. Conversely, some facilities not only bar children under age 19 as residents but also do not permit them even as overnight guests.

If it is important to you to live in a community where property ownership or occupancy is limited to older persons, you should inspect the deed or condominium declaration and bylaws to ensure that the age restrictions exist and are enforceable. If supportive services are important, you should be aware that there is rarely any guarantee that such services will continue to be provided in the future. Even the current recreational facilities may not be maintained or provided in the future.

If the age-restricted property is rented, the landlord can choose the nature of the age restrictions. Unless it is part of the written lease, a landlord's promise to operate an age-restricted facility is not enforceable. Under the Statute of Frauds, oral promises regarding property are normally not enforceable, although applicability of the Statute of Frauds varies according to state law. The general rule, however, is that oral promises or representations regarding rental property are not enforceable. The provisions of the written lease determine the obligations of the landlord.

Also keep in mind that the landlord of age-restricted housing has no legal obligation to provide services or facilities that serve the needs of older persons. Consequently, you should note carefully what services, if any, are provided and whether the landlord has promised in writing to continue to provide those services. Also pay close attention to the physical nature of the building. For example, a few stairs leading up to an apartment may prove difficult or impossible for a resident suffering from arthritis. If you wish to leave before the end of the lease term, even for medical reasons, you may be financially responsible for the remaining term of the lease. The lease provisions will determine whether you can sublease your unit to someone else for the remainder of the lease. Even if subleasing is permitted, you will have to rent to someone who meets the facility's age restrictions.

Varieties of Retirement Housing

Planned Communities

Many seniors are attracted to planned communities, which are collections of houses or townhouses controlled by a homeowners association. The primary purpose of the homeowners association is to enforce the community's uniform standards and to assess fees for the upkeep and maintenance of the common areas, including recreational facilities such as tennis courts, exercise facilities, and swimming pools. There are usually strict rules about the appearance and use of properties in the community. Planned communities generally appeal to those who value uniformity of appearance, quality of design and construction, and standards for use and maintenance. They are often gated and limit access to provide increased security for their residents.

The uniformity of design and maintenance and the right to impose fees result from legal land use controls known as easements and covenants. These restrictions are said to "run with the land," meaning that they are enforceable against the original owner and also against subsequent purchasers. Easements usually establish rights-of-way for access, common area use, parking, and utilities. Covenants are restrictions that typically govern design features and the type of structures that can be built. They are also used to prevent certain actions, such as subdividing lots, and even may prohibit what the community considers to be eyesores, such as satellite dishes, fences, and utility sheds. Covenants also subject properties to control by the homeowners association and to certain payment obligations, such as maintenance fees.

If you are considering the purchase of a house or condominium in a planned community, you should ask to examine the community's Declaration of Restrictive Covenants. All easements and covenants that benefit or restrict use of the property either will appear directly in the property's deed or the deed will likely reference another document where the easements and covenants are described. At the time you purchase the property, you are also considered to be "on notice" of any easements and restrictions that have been properly recorded in the property's "chain of title" regardless of whether those restrictions appear in your individual deed. The chain of title is made up of all of the recorded deeds and agreements that affect the property.

It is generally too late when you accept a deed at closing to decide that you no longer want the property because of certain easements or covenants. You should carefully consider such restrictions before you sign the purchase agreement or include in the purchase agreement a contingency that allows you a reasonable amount of time to review the restrictions and change your mind about the purchase. If you request a title report, it will identify all of the important documents that affect the property's chain of title, but you must still read the contents of those documents to learn about the restrictions. Before you sign anything, you should consider having a lawyer review these documents and the terms of the proposed purchase agreement if you are uncertain about your rights and responsibilities.

Covenants in planned communities can generally be enforced by any other property owner in the community or by the homeowners association. Most covenants can be eliminated only upon the agreement of all of the parties who have a right to enforce the covenant, typically all landowners in the development. For example, suppose all the lots are subject to a covenant that requires houses to be two stories tall. Several years after the opening of the development, the final vacant lot is sold. The new owner wishes to build a one-story house, which would not be permitted by the covenant. If all the other property owners agree to waive their right to enforce the covenant, the new lot owner will be able to build a one-story house. But if only one other property owner objects, the new lot owner will have to build a two-story house.

In some communities, the initial covenants create authority in the homeowners association, or in a certain percentage of the property owners, to make decisions that will bind all property owners in the development. This authority may include the power to terminate existing covenants or to create new ones. It is therefore important that you consider whether this method of decisionmaking is acceptable to you and whether your opinions are likely to be shared by a majority of your neighbors.

In addition to easements and covenants that directly affect the use of individual properties in a planned community, residents are usually subject to other rules created by the homeowners association. Although most of the rules center on the use of the common areas, the association may have authority to regulate use of individual properties or units. For example, the association may be able to limit who may enter the grounds of the community. This in turn might potentially limit the kind and frequency of services that can be brought to your home. If you might require in-home assistance, it is best to learn whether the association has any rules that might prohibit access to that type of service provider. Even if the association has no rules at present that would cause a conflict, does the association have the power to enact such rules in the future?

Condominiums. Many seniors move to condominiums where they still have the economic advantages of home ownership but are spared most maintenance and repair problems. Although condominiums do have many advantages, they represent a form of property ownership with unique rights and responsibilities.

Ownership. The basis of a condominium is a registered corporation that is operated by the condominium unit owners, who own an individual interest in an apartment or a townhouse and a shared interest in the common areas, such as the land, parking areas, elevators, stairways, and recreational areas. The unit owners own and are responsible for everything within their units, but the common, shared ownership areas, including central furnaces or other mechanical equipment, are supported by a monthly maintenance fee paid by each unit owner.

The condominium is operated under a master deed, called the Declaration of Condominium, that contains a description of the land and the other common elements, a list of the individual units, and a description of how the corporation or association is governed. The unit owners each have a deed that shows ownership of their individual units and joint ownership of the common areas and that subjects them to the provisions of the declaration, the rules of the unit owners association, and all restrictions, covenants, and easements contained in the master deed. Ongoing governance of the condominium is by a unit owners association, whose leadership is selected by the unit owners.

Condominium Governance. Initially, the developer of the condominium owns all the units and the common areas. But after a certain number of the units are sold, the unit owners organize a unit owners association that elects a board of directors, which in turn manages the property, assesses the monthly common area maintenance fee, and adopts rules and regulations for the operation of the condominium. The rights and duties of the board of directors are stated in the Declaration of the Condominium and include operating the commonly owned property, such as the common entry and the elevator or stairs leading to the units.

The declaration states the voting power of each unit (which is usually one vote for each unit); the percentage of unit owners required to approve amendments to the declaration (subject to state law requirements); the rules for electing a board of directors and officers; and what kinds of bylaws may be adopted by the board and what bylaws must be approved by the unit owners. Although the votes of a majority or supermajority of unit owners is usually all that is needed to govern, some decisions, such as increasing the number of units or selling common property, may be subject to state laws that require unanimous consent of the unit owners.

If you are considering the purchase of a condominium, you should carefully examine the declaration and the condominium bylaws to see whether you can live with the various restrictions. Special attention should be paid to any rights of the board of directors to limit or regulate the use of individual units. For example, you should be sure that nothing in the condominium rules will prohibit in-home care if it is eventually needed.

The unit owners association assesses a monthly fee upon all unit owners for the repair, maintenance, and property taxes on the common areas. Unit owners are responsible for their share of the assessment even if they do not use the common area. For example, even if you never use a commonly owned tennis court, you will still be responsible for helping to pay for the court maintenance and repair. In addition to paying for normal maintenance, members can be assessed by the board of directors for special repairs such as fixing the roof or replacing the furnace. The condominium declaration may require a vote by a supermajority to authorize a special assessment to pay for unusual or major repairs.

Failure to pay an assessment will result in a lien against the unit, which is a legal obligation to pay the assessment from the sale proceeds if the unit is sold. A lien may become attached to the property despite valid claims by the unit owner that the condominium association did not provide the level of service called for in the declaration or bylaws. If the unit is sold without payment of the assessment and release of the lien, the new purchaser's interest in the unit will be subject to the lien. Consequently, when purchasing a condominium unit, you should examine the title report to identify any outstanding liens and obtain an agreement from the seller that such liens will be satisfied on or before closing of the sale.

Architectural control restrictions are common with condominiums. These generally restrict external changes to the unit. Internal changes rarely need approval. Some modifications, such as satellite dishes or changes to the windows, may be prohibited. In contrast, modest changes may be permitted, but only with the approval of the board of directors. Some larger condominiums have an architectural review board that must approve significant modifications of the individual units that are visible from the street. Even some internal modifications may need approval, particularly if they result in a change to the exterior of the unit. You should not purchase a condominium expecting to change its appearance without first obtaining the assurance of the board of directors that it will not interfere with the proposed alteration.

If a unit owner's request to modify the exterior is refused, the unit owner can sue, but she or he will probably lose because courts are reluctant to overrule subjective decisions about the appearance of property. If the board does not consistently enforce its rules, however, the unit owner may win.

Pets. The issue of pets can be very controversial in a condominium setting. Some condominiums have no policy; residents are free to own pets as they see fit. More commonly, condominiums restrict the number of pets per unit and sometimes the kind of pet, such as prohibiting cats or dogs but permitting birds and fish. Other condominiums limit the size of dogs by pounds or height. Some only forbid "dangerous" animals, such as snakes.

Before buying a condominium, you should ask about the rule on pets. Even if you have no pets, it is important to know whether the other unit owners are permitted to own them. Seeing dogs or cats on the premises does not necessarily mean that the condominium permits them. Such pets may have been grandfathered in when the condominium adopted restrictions prohibiting new dogs or cats. Also consider that if the condominium forbids all pets, or all cats and dogs, such a prohibition might make the condominium less attractive to buyers when the time comes to sell it. Condominium pet restrictions are frequently litigated, but usually courts uphold the restrictions so long as they are consistently applied.

Liability Issues. State law determines the potential liability of condominium owners. Condominium owners, if negligent, are liable for injuries to guests that occur in their unit. They may also be liable for injuries to individuals that happen in the common areas. Because of the potential for liability, a unit owner should buy adequate liability insurance and insist that the condominium association carry high-limit liability insurance for the common areas as well as liability insurance to protect board members, officers, and others against claims arising from their acts on behalf of the association.

Limits on Lease or Sale. Some condominiums have restrictions on the sale of a unit, but that is unusual. More common are limits on leasing a unit. Some even prohibit altogether the renting of units. If you are purchasing a unit for seasonal residence, it may be important to you to rent the unit when you are not using it. Or if you need to sell the unit, but the real estate market is slow, you may wish to rent the unit until the market improves. Consequently, it is a good idea to inquire about leasing policies before purchasing a condominium unit.

Cooperatives. Cooperatives, although seemingly similar to condominiums, are in fact quite different. The most significant difference is that a condominium unit owner actually owns the unit but the occupant of a cooperative unit does not. Rather, a resident in a cooperative development owns shares in the cooperative, which in turn owns all the units. Ownership of the shares gives the shareholder exclusive possession of a particular apartment unit, but that possession is subject to all of the rules in the cooperative shareholders agreement.

A board of directors makes most of the important decisions for the cooperative, including decisions about who may purchase shares of the cooperative. Thus, if you live in a cooperative and want to move, you can sell your shares only with the approval of the board of directors. The board can withhold consent to transfer shares for any reason it chooses so long as it is not a legally prohibited reason such as race, religion, or sex. For example, boards have rejected potential shareholders on reasonable bases, such as a poor credit rating, as well as on bases that some would view as unreasonable, such as the potential shareholder's political affiliation or profession. Most cooperatives insist that the buyer pay cash for shares and will not approve the sale of shares financed by a mortgage. As a result, a cooperative member may find that it takes longer to dispose of a cooperative unit than other forms of housing.

Mobile and Manufactured Homes. Many seniors live in mobile and manufactured homes because of the cost savings. By lowering the cost of their housing, the owners have more disposable income to spend on other needs. Thanks to the federal Manufactured Home Construction and Safety Standards (42 U.S.C. §§5401 *et seq.*), which mandate specifications for strength, durability, fire and wind resistance, and energy efficiency, today's manufactured houses are competitive in construction with traditional houses. Despite improvements in quality, mobile and manufactured homes may not be available in all areas due to restrictive zoning laws.

There are some significant differences between manufactured and mobile homes. A manufactured house looks very much like a traditional house, though it costs less to build because it features walls built offsite and may have metal where a traditional house would have wood. The owner of a manufactured home, like the owner of a traditional home, generally owns the land on which the house is located. In contrast, mobile home owners, whose homes are located in a mobile home park, usually do not own the land upon which their homes are located. Rather, they rent the lot, which can create a problem if they want to relocate.

The high cost of moving a mobile home generally means that if the owner wants to move, he or she must sell the mobile home to someone who will take over the lease of the lot on which it is located. Some landlords try to restrict such sales with lease clauses that either force removal of the mobile home or result in its sale at a bargain price to the landlord. To protect mobile home owners, many states have laws overriding such restrictions. State laws may also limit the grounds on which a landlord can evict a mobile home park tenant as a check-and-balance on landlords using eviction to force a sale of the mobile home.

Although mobile homes are generally less costly than traditional or other manufactured houses, financing a mobile home can be difficult because mortgages are usually shorter in duration and carry a higher interest rate. Casualty insurance may also be more costly in relation to the value of the home, typically 25 to 30 percent higher. However, in many jurisdictions, a mobile home is classified as personal property and so is not subject to local property taxes. Despite some of these issues, the overall cost savings make mobile homes an attractive option for low-income seniors.

Supportive Housing

Many older seniors find that they need daily assistance. Fortunately, supportive housing—that is, housing that offers assistance inside the home—is available in a variety of forms and at a range of prices.

Congregate Housing

"Congregate housing" is a term used to describe a variety of housing that combines age restrictions with some nonmedical services. Usually constructed in the form of apartments or condominiums, it is designed for individuals capable of independent living. The individual units are supplemented with some common areas, such as a library, card rooms, and, perhaps, a dining room. Whether a condominium or rental facility, the monthly fee will include the cost of providing limited in-unit housekeeping services. Even though the facility may have a dining room, it may not serve three meals a day. Even the evening meal may be optional, although some congregate housing facilities mandate the evening meal to support the cost of a dining facility.

A monthly fee pays for all repair and maintenance of both the common areas and the individual units. Housekeeping, including a change of bed linens and cleaning of the unit, is usually also provided. The facility will not provide medical monitoring or assistance, nor will the facility provide personal in-unit care. Congregate housing is not a viable option if you need daily, in-unit care.

For some seniors, congregate housing is attractive because it is age restricted; it offers housekeeping, some recreational facilities, and a sense of community; and it does not have the costs of additional supportive services. They assume that if personal care or medical services are later needed, they will move to a facility that will meet that need. In particular, congregate housing developments attract many seniors who do not want to move into "elderly housing" before they need the kind of personal and limited medical care offered in an assisted living facility. If you are considering congregate housing, you should investigate its financial stability. Competitive pressures have resulted in some of these facilities going into bankruptcy.

Assisted Living Facilities

An assisted living facility (ALF), as opposed to congregate living, is for individuals who need personal assistance in addition to the conveniences of congregate living. The need for personal assistance may result from physical infirmities, memory difficulties, or both. Separately or combined, mental and physical problems are the reason that millions of older seniors live in housing that provides supportive personal care and some medical assistance. Whereas some seniors are ill enough to need nursing home care, most do not. Today, more than 80 percent of ALF residents are women with an average age near 80.

In the past, assisted living was more commonly known as board and care homes, personal care homes, or retirement homes. In some states, assisted living is merely a board and care home with a new name. Other states, however, have adopted regulations that distinguish ALFs from board and care homes, with ALFs being licensed to care for individuals who need personal care and modest medical supervision. ALFs can also serve as temporary posthospitalization residences or provide short-term respite care for families who care for an older person at home.

ALFs vary from state to state in response to state regulations. Generally, however, they feature individual or shared studio apartments and provide three meals a day served in a common dining area, as well as housekeeping services, in-unit personal care as needed, and medication management. The facility provides round-the-clock staff and supervision, in-room emergency call systems, and, usually, some limited social and recreational activities. Some ALFs also provide transportation services for shopping and medical appointments.

The goal of assisted living is to provide a level of care that will delay the need to move to a more institutionalized and expensive nursing home. For many frail elderly, or those who have dementia but are otherwise healthy, assisted living is a safe, affordable alternative to living alone. Those with mild to moderate dementia often live in a special section of an assisted living facility so that they can be monitored and prevented from wandering away from the facility.

Although assisted living is designed for seniors with personal care needs, the distinction between personal care and medical care is an important one. An ALF is a personal care provider, not a medical provider. Residents must be able to get out of bed and to the dining room. State assisted living regulations usually prevent ALFs from admitting bedfast individuals because they require a degree of health care that can be provided only in a licensed nursing home. Some state laws permit an assisted living facility to continue to house residents who become bedfast if a physician will certify that they are not in need of skilled nursing care.

Most ALF residents are unable to perform some activities of daily living (ADLs). Although there is no formal, legal definition of ADLs, the term is usually meant to refer to

- bathing
- toileting
- eating
- dressing
- ambulating (getting out of a chair or bed without assistance)

An individual who cannot perform one of these tasks without assistance is said to have an ADL deficit and is in need of custodial care as opposed to skilled nursing, which provides medical care.

Another measure of a person's capabilities for self care are the instrumental activities of daily living (IADLs), which include going grocery shopping, using a telephone, cleaning a house, and paying bills. Some assisted living residents have no ADL deficits but move into the facility because they cannot perform IADLs. For example, they may have very poor vision and so are unable to navigate in the larger world.

The goal of an assisted living facility is to provide a safe and supportive environment that includes meals and assistance with bathing, grooming, and dressing. The facility monitors the individual's health and will likely have a nurse on its staff. It will have procedures to ensure that residents regularly take their medications. Some facilities also provide or contract for Medicare-reimbursed home health or rehabilitative care.

Residents of assisted living sign an admission contract. The resident agrees to pay the daily or monthly cost of care in exchange for the facility agreeing to provide room and board and specified personal care. Prior to entering the facility, the individual may be required to submit to a physical examination. Individuals who are too sick or who have more advanced dementia will not be admitted because the facility is not licensed to provide the level of care that they need. Some ALFs also charge an "entrance fee" that is often equivalent to two months rent and nonrefundable. Admission contracts vary but generally contain the following:

- date of initial occupancy
- identification of the unit to be occupied
- specification of who provides the room furnishings (usually the resident)
- a list of the services that the facility will provide (it may also list additional services that can be purchased)
- the monthly fee and any security deposit (including the right of the ALF to raise the fee)
- the right of the resident to return to the room after a period of hospitalization
- the conditions under which the facility can move (such as to a dementia ward) or evict the resident

Because state regulation of assisted living facilities is minimal, it is important that you carefully review the admission contract. Many contracts give the ALF management broad discretion to determine whether you meet the requirements for continued residence in the facility. Consider, for example, a situation in which you have suffered a moderate stroke. Your doctor believes that with speech and physical therapy you will have a full recovery; however, that may take three to four months to achieve. During that period, will the ALF allow caregivers to assist you in your room or apartment? If not, do you have the right to pay to keep your apartment available while you recover somewhere else? Could you afford to do this? Some ALFs are associated with nursing homes and require residents to move to the nursing home when they no longer meet the standards for semi-independent living in the ALF.

The lack of protection against the ALF management terminating your right to remain in the facility, or to return after a hospital stay, is one of the disadvantages of assisted living. A few states have laws that give ALF residents some of the same protections as other tenants of rental housing have, but most do not. You should also keep in mind that a number of the in-home services that are available to seniors aging in place in their own residence (such as services provided through Medicaid waivers or the Area Agency on Aging) are not permitted in ALFs.

Residents of assisted living usually pay their own way. There is almost no public reimbursement of the cost of assisted living. A few states provide limited Medicaid waivers to help with the cost of assisted living. Most residents who run out of money must leave the facility. Many who do so move to a nursing home where they can qualify for Medicaid reimbursement. Most long-term care insurance pays benefits to residents of assisted living provided that they have difficulty performing at least two ADLs or they are cognitively impaired, such as having dementia.

Because seniors who live in assisted living often spend down a considerable amount of their assets doing so, they may have few financial options left if a temporary health crisis occurs. Often rehabilitation in a nursing home after a hospitalization event turns into permanent residence because of the lack of funds to reenter assisted living or obtain other independent or retirement housing. Therefore, before you leave your own residence to move to assisted living, ask yourself the following questions:

- How much help do I need?
- Can my home be modified to make living there easier?
- Can I hire the additional help that I need?
- How much would services in my home cost?
- If I move to assisted living, how long will I be able to afford to live there?

You should compare the costs of living in your own residence with the costs of living in an assisted living facility. Most seniors can purchase considerable services in their own home before the cost approaches the cost of assisted living.

Board and Care Homes

Board and care homes, also known as personal care or retirement homes, provide care for many seniors, particularly those with lower incomes. Even though such facilities vary greatly, they provide room, board, and some degree of personal care. A few house hundreds of residents. Others are merely older houses converted into a board and care home and have as few as three or four residents. It is estimated that there are fifty thousand licensed homes across the nation, with six hundred thousand or more residents.

Even though such homes are supposed to be licensed by the state and subject to periodic inspection, many smaller ones operate without a license. For example, a couple may merely take in older persons without bothering to obtain a state license. Typically, board and care homes are much less costly and provide fewer amenities than ALFs. In some states, board and care homes are licensed to care for individuals who require less personal care or assistance than do the residents of assisted living. Such board and care homes function more as boarding houses than as care facilities.

Some board and care homes are sponsored by nonprofit organizations or churches, but most are privately run, profit-seeking businesses. Most residents are private pay, but many states subsidize the cost of the very poor residents' care, sometimes augmenting the individual's monthly Supplemental Security Income (SSI) benefit (see Chapter 3 for general information about SSI eligibility).

Board and care homes are regulated by the state governments. If they house a significant number of SSI recipients, they are subject to federal requirements that the state establish and enforce minimum standards. However, because the penalty for failing to maintain these standards is reduction in the SSI payment to the resident, rather than a penalty on the noncompliant facility, the law is rarely enforced.

Continuing Care Retirement Communities

Continuing care retirement communities (CCRCs) provide three levels of housing: independent living, assisted living, and nursing home care. They advertise that once admitted, you will never have to leave to find appropriate care.

CCRCs are found in cities, suburbs, and rural areas. Some feature single-story townhouses, whereas others are high rises. Most have a central facility that contains the shared amenities, such as a dining room and recreational facilities. Usually, the assisted living units and the nursing home beds are also located there. A few CCRCs lack nursing home beds and contract for that care at offsite locations. CCRCs are operated by both for-profit and nonprofit entities. The nonprofit CCRCs are often affiliated with a religious organization. These facilities sometimes solicit charitable funds to help subsidize the monthly fee of lower-income residents or to pay for those who have run out of money.

Residents of CCRCs pay both a monthly residence fee, which can run from $3,000 to $6,000 per month, and an initial admission fee, which is usually $100,000 to $500,000. The initial admission fee may be refundable in diminishing amounts the longer the individual resides in the facility, or the resident may have the option of a smaller, nonrefundable admission fee. Obviously, CCRCs are not for the poor. To be admitted, you must provide financial proof that you will be able to afford the monthly fee now and as it rises in the future.

Most residents raise the money for the admission fee by the sale of their houses. A few CCRCs sell the independent living units to the residents, who in turn resell the unit when they leave it. The admission fee is a form of long-term care insurance that is purchased at the time of admission to the CCRC. It represents, in part, prepayment for health care that may be needed later. Generally, the monthly fee will not rise merely because the resident requires more assistance; however, some CCRCs do charge a somewhat higher fee if the resident requires skilled nursing care. The part of the admission fee that is prepayment for health care is deductible on the resident's federal income tax as a Section 213 medical deduction (I.R.C. §213[d]).

CCRCs only admit individuals capable of independent living and require a physical examination as proof of their ability to live in an independent living unit. The unit will be an unfurnished studio or one, two, or even three bedroom unit, which contains a small kitchen. The CCRC provides one meal a day in the common dining room as well as recreational and social opportunities. Most residents will own a car and experience the CCRC much as if they were living in an age-restricted apartment. But as they age, they will receive more supportive services. The individual will reside in the independent living unit until unable to do so because of mental or physical problems. At that time, the resident will move to an assisted living unit, which will be smaller, have no cooking facilities, and be located in the central building or part of the facility. Because residents are reluctant to move to the assisted living units, CCRCs often provide custodial care, such as help with dressing, in the independent living units, but they charge a daily service fee for doing so.

The monthly fee pays for the meal (or three meals if the resident is in assisted living or in the nursing home), all utilities, recreational facilities such as an indoor swimming pool, and the various services provided by the facility. Many CCRCs offer breakfast and lunch on a per-meal payment to those living independently.

CCRCs are regulated only by states except for their nursing homes, which must comply with federal regulations if they receive Medicare and Medicaid reimbursement. State regulation varies considerably. From a resident's standpoint, the market is the best regulator because a CCRC must appeal to individuals who have enough resources and income to have a choice as to where they seek long-term care. The biggest fear is that the CCRC will run into financial difficulties and not be able to provide the promised care. States try to protect residents by requiring CCRCs to place a portion of the admission fee into an escrow or other protected account. Before signing the contract of admission to a CCRC, you should insist on reviewing a financial statement for the CCRC to assess its financial stability. A CCRC may also be subject to state laws that govern providers of assisted living at least as to the CCRC's assisted living units.

Problems often arise when the CCRC wants to move the resident from an independent living unit to assisted living. Residents are naturally resistant to such a move because they will be moved into a smaller unit, have less privacy, and lose their kitchen. The resident may suspect that part of the motive for the move is the desire of the CCRC to release or sell the vacated independent living unit. Unfortunately for the resident, the contract of admission will permit the CCRC to move the resident to assisted living or to the nursing home without the resident's consent.

The real protection for the resident is the CCRC's fear of bad publicity should the resident create a fuss about the move. Usually, the CCRC will negotiate with a reluctant resident and gradually convince the resident and the resident's family that a move is necessary because of the resident's declining health. Occasionally, a resident will become so difficult to deal with—possibly because of dementia—that the CCRC will evict him or her. The contract of admission usually permits this. The resident's only recourse is to claim that the illness is not severe enough to trigger the eviction conditions as specified in the admission contract. The resident can also claim that eviction would violate the federal Fair Housing Act (42 U.S.C. §§3601 *et seq.*) or the federal Rehabilitation Act (29 U.S.C. §§701 *et seq.*), which prohibits a federally funded state program from discriminating against a handicapped individual solely by reason of the handicap.

Nursing Homes

More than 1.6 million, or about 4.5 percent of Americans age 65 or older live in a nursing home. Of those age 85 or older, about 12 percent of the men and 21 percent of the women live in a nursing home. The length of stay in nursing homes varies considerably. Some residents stay only a short time while they recover from a temporary health crisis for which they were hospitalized. Some, the very ill, die soon after they enter the facility. For other seniors, particularly those with dementia, the stay in a nursing home can extend for years until finally ended by death. In the past twenty years, however, both the percentage of seniors in a nursing home and the length of the average stay have dropped. In part this is a reflection of the popularity of assisted living, and in part the lower numbers reflect the relatively improved health of seniors.

Federal law defines "nursing home" as an institution that provides skilled nursing care or rehabilitation services for injured, disabled, or sick persons as well as custodial care, which is defined as health-related care and services above the level of room and board. Such care is expensive. The average monthly cost of a nursing home runs from $5,000 to more than $8,000 a month. The cost of labor is usually the main reason for the extreme differences in cost.

Nursing homes, while necessary, are usually viewed negatively as institutions that take away an individual's autonomy, privacy, and independence. Residents usually share a room and have a set schedule for meals, showers, and activities. Many residents are bedridden, vulnerable, and very dependent on the staff. Nevertheless, for many, only a nursing home offers the needed combination of custodial and skilled nursing care. In response to complaints about their institutional nature, some nursing homes are making renovations to be more homelike, such as replacing long hospital-like corridors with clusters of rooms.

Because almost all nursing homes participate in Medicare and Medicaid, they are subject to federal laws and regulations, the result of which is that most nursing home operations are fairly similar. Medicare, the federal program of subsidized health care for those age 65 and older, reimburses only skilled nursing care. The Medicare skilled nursing benefit is available only for nursing home care immediately following a hospital stay of at least three continuous days (not counting the day of discharge) and if recommended by a physician. When these conditions are met, Medicare will pay for the following:

- physician's services
- twenty-four-hour nursing services
- room and board, including specialized dietary services
- rehabilitative services such as speech, physical, or occupational therapy
- drugs supervised by a pharmacist and delivered by a nurse
- laboratory and diagnostic services
- medically related social services
- appropriate resident activities

Medicare pays for nursing home care as a means of encouraging patients to leave very expensive hospitals and move into relatively affordable nursing homes. The program was not intended to reimburse long-term care and so pays for only one hundred days of skilled nursing home care. After the first twenty days, the resident has a co-pay, which in 2010 was $137.50 per day. The amount is adjusted annually.

More than one-half of all nursing home costs are paid for by Medicaid, a federal-state program based on financial need that will pay for the cost of a nursing home for as long as it is needed (see Chapter 6 for general information on Medicaid eligibility). Although Medicaid has no co-pay, in essence it requires nursing home residents to exhaust nearly all of their assets and to apply all of their income to the cost of the nursing home care before Medicaid will begin to reimburse the cost of care. Medicaid pays for both skilled and custodial care. Like Medicare, Medicaid also requires a physician's order for care, but unlike Medicare, it does not require any period of prior hospitalization.

Regulation

Nursing homes are heavily regulated by both the federal and state governments. Every nursing home needs a state-issued license to operate. The federal government does not license nursing homes, but nursing homes must take care to comply with federal requirements under the Medicaid and Medicare programs or risk loss of funding. Federal regulations give residents detailed rights that must be observed by nursing homes that participate in Medicare or Medicaid. (Residents' rights are found in the Code of Federal Regulations, 42 C.F.R. §483.10.) A few nursing homes do not accept Medicare or Medicaid and so are not subject to federal law, but state licensing requirements generally mirror the federal rules so that all nursing homes are essentially subject to the same requirements. In addition, nursing homes are also subject to federal and state civil rights laws, consumer protection statutes, and state common-law tort and contract remedies.

The nursing home medical supervisor is responsible for the coordination, adequacy, and appropriateness of resident care. Federal law requires that a physician must see each resident in a nursing home at least once every thirty days during the first ninety days of residence and at least once every sixty days thereafter (42 C.F.R. §483.40[c][1]). New residents must be given a comprehensive assessment fourteen days after admission, which must be updated once a year to ensure that the nursing home is appropriate for their needs (42 C.F.R. §483.20[b][2]).

Nursing homes must also assess residents at least every three months by using a state-approved review procedure (42 C.F.R. §483.20[c]). The initial assessment is used to create an individual, written care plan that details the necessary treatment and rehabilitation efforts to be provided to the resident. If the resident's condition changes significantly, there must be a new comprehensive assessment within fourteen days (42 C.F.R. §483.20[b][2]). The assessments, signed by a registered nurse, are to be used to monitor, develop, review, and revise the resident's care plan. Families of new residents should insist upon obtaining a copy of the assessments and the care plan so that they can monitor whether the facility is carrying out its obligations under the plan.

Contracts of Admission. A new resident of a nursing home is required to sign a contract of admission. If the resident is mentally incapacitated, the individual's guardian or family member will sign the agreement. Depending on state law, a nursing home may have some discretion about whom it admits. Most prefer not to admit mentally ill or mentally retarded individuals and so use a preadmission screening to identify individuals whom they are not legally required to admit. Note that dementia is not grounds for an admission refusal.

Many nursing homes prefer private pay residents as opposed to those who are paid for by Medicaid because the nursing home typically charges a higher private pay daily rate than Medicaid is willing to pay. Medicaid is notorious for paying a low daily rate—so low that a nursing home cannot operate if every resident is Medicaid reimbursed. Whether a nursing home can refuse a Medicaid patient, or one who is likely to become a Medicaid patient, depends upon state law.

As a practical matter, most nursing homes probably give admission preference to private pay residents. Some state laws prevent the nursing home from giving preference to private pay patients in its admissions policy, and some states require that a certain percentage of the patients admitted be Medicaid patients. Once admitted, however, no resident can be prevented from seeking and accepting Medicaid reimbursement (42 C.F.R. §483.12[d][1][i] and [ii]).

Federal law also prohibits Medicare- or Medicaid-reimbursed nursing homes from requiring a third party to guarantee payment as a condition of admission (42 C.F.R. §483.12[d][2]). Nevertheless, many nursing homes do attempt to induce family members to sign the admission contract as a responsible party who agrees to pay the nursing home in the event that the resident cannot and is not eligible for Medicaid. These so-called responsible party agreements may not be enforceable, although state law differs. The best advice is to refuse to sign such an agreement.

Transfers and Discharges. Residents are protected under federal and state laws against unwarranted transfers and discharges. These laws apply even when there are contrary terms in the nursing home admission contract. Before any transfer or discharge, the facility must notify the resident, a family member, or guardian at least thirty days in advance and explain the reasons for the move (42 C.F.R. §483.12[a][5][i]). Under federal law, a resident can be transferred only for medical reasons, for the welfare of the resident, for the welfare of other residents, for nonpayment, or because the facility is ceasing to operate (42 C.F.R. §483.12[a][2]). The advance notice of thirty days is inapplicable if one of the following conditions applies:

- The transfer is necessary for the health or safety of residents.
- The resident's health has improved enough that the resident no longer qualifies for nursing home care.
- The resident's urgent medical needs require a more immediate transfer (42 C.F.R. §483.12[a][5][ii]).

Before discharging a resident, the nursing home must create a postdischarge plan of care (42 C.F.R. §483.20[l][3]). If a resident goes to a hospital, the nursing home must explain its bed-hold policy, that is, the resident's right to return (42 C.F.R. §483.12[b]). When transferring or discharging residents, a nursing home must treat all of them alike regardless of whether they pay for their own care or their care is paid for by Medicare or Medicaid (42 C.F.R. §483.12[c]).

Federal Nursing Home Reform Act. The most important source of resident rights is the federal Nursing Home Reform Act, which applies to all nursing homes that accept Medicare or Medicaid (42 U.S.C. §1395i-3 [Medicare]; 42 U.S.C. §1396r [Medicaid]). The act, part of the Omnibus Budget Reconciliation Act of 1987 (Pub. L. No. 100-203, 101 Stat. 1330), requires that nursing homes must "promote maintenance or enhancement of the quality of life of each resident" (42 U.S.C. §1395i-3[b][1][A] [Medicare]; 42 U.S.C. §1396r[b][1][A] [Medicaid]). Unfortunately, an individual resident cannot sue to enforce the act, which is enforceable only by the state or federal government. Nevertheless, the act can be used to define the quality-of-care standard that should be expected of nursing homes.

The act's requirements are explained in the Code of Federal Regulations beginning at 42 C.F.R. §483. These regulations require that at the time of admission to the facility, the nursing home must tell a resident about the resident's rights and also provide the resident with a written copy of those rights (42 C.F.R. §483.10[b]). These rights include the following:

- *Freedom of choice*: Residents have a right to choose their own doctor and to help plan their care and treatment decisions.
- *Freedom from restraints and abuse*: Residents have a right to be free of chemical and physical restraints except to ensure their physical safety or that of other residents, and then only upon a physician's written order specifying the duration and circumstances of the restraint.
- *Privacy*: Residents have a right to privacy as to their medical treatment, written and telephonic communications, visits, and meetings with their families.
- *Confidentiality*: All personal and clinical records of residents must be kept confidential. A resident or a resident's legal representative has a right to access current records within twenty-four hours of making such a request.
- *Accommodation of individual needs*: Residents have a right to care that meets their individual needs.
- *Personal items*: Residents have a right to personal items, including furniture, clothing, and decorations.
- *Grievances*: Residents have a right to voice grievances about their treatment or care without fear of retaliation.
- *Participation in groups and other activities*: Residents have a right to participate in resident groups and social, religious, and community activities. Families of residents have the right to meet together in the facility.
- *Examination of survey results*: Residents have a right to the official survey results of a nursing home. The facility must post a notice of the availability of the survey.
- *Access and visitation rights*: Residents have a right to see governmental representatives, their individual physicians, the state's long-term care ombudsman, and anyone who provides health, social, legal, or other services to residents.

Nursing homes cannot charge residents for items that are paid for by Medicare or Medicaid, including routine personal hygiene items such as soap, razors, toothbrushes, tissues, deodorants, dental care items, incontinence care supplies, and over-the-counter drugs (42 C.F.R. §483.10[c][8][i]). The nursing home, however, can charge for in-room telephones, televisions, and radios; cosmetic and grooming items not paid for by Medicare or Medicaid; flowers and plants; and special food even if required by dietary or medical needs (42 C.F.R. §483.10[c][8][ii]). Medicare and Medicaid pay only for a shared room unless a private room is needed for a therapeutic reason such as isolation for infection control. A resident who wants a private room must pay the additional daily fee.

Theft and loss of residents' personal property and money are common problems. Federal law requires nursing homes to safeguard and account for residents' funds and maintain a written record of all financial transactions involving the personal funds of a resident that were deposited with the facility (42 C.F.R. §483.10[c]). Any resident funds in excess of $50 must be deposited into an interest-bearing account. Within thirty days of the resident's death, the facility must give the resident's personal funds to the administrator of the resident's estate and provide a final accounting.

State Ombudsman

Federal funding is provided to each state for the purpose of operating a Long-Term Care Ombudsman Office, the duty of which is to identify, investigate, and resolve complaints made by nursing home residents or others on their behalf (42 U.S.C. §3058g). The ombudsman investigates nursing homes to assure that they are providing proper care for their residents and may investigate other providers of long-term care services, as well as public health and social service agencies. If necessary, the ombudsman can represent residents before governmental agencies and is also expected to help develop citizen organizations that promote residents' rights. Anyone can contact the state Long-Term Care Ombudsman to register complaints or concern about the care provided by a nursing home.

Nursing Home Liability

Nursing home residents and their families are increasingly suing nursing homes and their staffs when the resident receives inadequate care, is injured, or dies due to a lack of proper care. Whereas in some instances the harm suffered by the resident may subject the nursing home or its employees to criminal liability, more common are civil lawsuits. These suits may be brought by the resident or the resident's family based on breach of the nursing home admission contract or on wrongful conduct known under the law as a "tort." Torts are categorized either as "intentional" or as "negligence." Nursing homes may be liable for intentional torts such as assault, battery, and false imprisonment or for the negligence of their staff. Absent contrary state law, the employer is liable for the personal injury or property damage, loss, or theft, whether intentional or negligent, caused by its employees.

Intentional Torts. Residents often sue claiming that they were the victims of harmful threats or contact that are known under the law as the intentional torts of assault and battery. Assault is defined as intentionally acting in a manner designed to cause a harmful or offensive contact or to create the fear of such contact. For example, throwing a tray toward a resident but missing her is an assault. Even a mere threat, such as "Eat or I'll slap you," can be an assault if it puts the victim in reasonable fear of imminent harmful or offensive contact.

Battery is an intentional harmful or offensive contact. It includes hitting, kissing, or striking the resident with an object. A battery occurs whenever the contact would be offensive to a reasonable person, though the victim does not need to be aware of the offensive touching. For example, fondling a sleeping resident is a battery.

There is also the tort of intentional infliction of emotional distress, defined as intentional or reckless acts of extreme or outrageous conduct that cause severe mental distress. One family member successfully sued for the intentional infliction of emotional distress when her 98-year-old mother was intentionally and maliciously hidden from her on three separate occasions when she came to visit her at the nursing home (*Miller v. Currie*, 50 F.3d 373 [6th Cir. 1995]).

Negligence. Negligence consists of failing to provide reasonable care to a resident. To bring a successful negligence case, the person claiming negligence must show that there was a duty of care, that the nursing home breached that duty, that the resident was injured, and that the injury was caused by the breach of duty. Most residents who claim that a nursing home acted negligently will have to prove that the facility failed to meet the proper standard of care and that this failure led to the resident's injuries. For example, when a resident suffers injuries from a fall, which is the most common basis for a negligence claim, liability is not established merely because the resident fell and was injured. The plaintiff must prove that the fall was the result of negligent care such as the failure of the nursing home to provide adequate supervision, failure to respond promptly to a call button, or failure to instruct the staff on how to prevent falls.

There are some exceptions to the need to provide proof of causation. Sometimes the existence of the injury itself is sufficient to prove negligence. For example, severe, infected bedsores or burns may be enough to establish what is known as a "prima facie" case of negligence by the nursing home. A prima facie case simply means that the facts are enough "on first appearance" to establish the elements. When the court finds that the severity of the injuries constitute a prima facie case, the burden shifts to the nursing home to bring forward contradictory evidence that it did not breach its duty of care.

Another exception to the need to produce proof of causation is the doctrine of *res ipsa loquitur* ("The thing speaks for itself"). Under this doctrine, the causation requirement is met by showing that when the resident was injured, the nursing home had exclusive control over the person or thing that injured the plaintiff and that the injury could not have occurred unless the nursing home was negligent. For example, the doctrine was applied in a case where a resident died when the respirator that was keeping her alive inexplicably stopped functioning (*Redfield v. Beverly Health & Rehabilitation Services, Inc.,* 42 S.W.3d 703 [Mo. Ct. App. 2001]). The respirator was under the exclusive control of the nursing home, and its stoppage was not something that would have occurred if the nursing home had exercised due care. Consequently, the court held that a jury could find that the nursing home had been negligent without specific proof of how the nursing home was negligent.

Even apart from what might be specified in the admission contract, every nursing home owes its residents a professional standard of care—typically defined as the level of care and skill used by other facilities in the community. The care must meet the needs of the resident in light of the resident's condition. What makes nursing home litigation difficult is that most residents are already suffering some type of serious physical ailment when they are admitted to the nursing home. Nursing homes often argue in defense of a negligence action that the resident's poor health upon admission was the cause of the resident's subsequent injury or poor condition rather than negligent care by the nursing home. For example, if a resident falls and breaks a hip, the nursing home may claim that despite its adequate supervision of the resident, his poor health led to his fall.

In some states, a lawsuit against a nursing home is considered a claim for medical malpractice, and so testimony by an expert witness is required. Also, there is usually a relatively short statute of limitations—the period of time in which to bring a claim after the harm has occurred—for malpractice actions. To avoid having the claim classified as a medical malpractice action, some residents have successfully sued under state consumer protection laws such as unfair trade practices laws.

Contract of Admission. Nursing home residents may also recover by claiming that the nursing home failed to provide the level of care promised in the contract of admission. Breach of contract, misrepresentation, fraud, and breach of implied warranties are all legitimate grounds for a lawsuit. However, most contract claims against nursing homes fail because the nursing home is careful to write the contract in a manner that favors the facility.

Mandatory Arbitration. Increasingly, nursing home contracts of admission require the resident to submit any potential lawsuit to mandatory arbitration and to agree to limits on possible damage awards. Although a few state courts have held such clauses to be unenforceable (*Bruner v. Timberlane Manor Ltd. P'ship,* 155 P.3d 16 [Okla. 2006]), the trend is to uphold them.[3]

As a result, an injured resident will not be able to sue in civil court but will have to submit the claim to arbitration and be content with limits on available damages, such as caps on awards for pain and suffering, and no punitive damages.

Choosing a Nursing Home

Although the operating standards for nursing homes are very similar community to community and state to state, the actual quality of life within a nursing home may vary greatly among facilities. This is due in large part to the philosophy of the nursing home management and the quantity and quality of its staff. So how can you make a good choice when it comes to a nursing home for yourself or someone else?

Making an informed decision about a nursing home involves doing some background investigation as well as spending time visiting facilities and asking questions. The federal government has a website called Nursing Home Compare, which provides detailed information about the quality of all nursing homes that are certified to receive Medicare and Medicaid funds. You can search nursing homes by state, county, or closeness to your location using your city name or zip code. If you know the name of a particular nursing home, you can also use the name as a way to access information. On this website there is also a link to a list of nursing homes that have a record of persistently poor performances and thus have been selected for more frequent inspections and monitoring.

Keep in mind that all Medicare- and Medicaid-certified nursing homes are subject to an annual review process called a "survey." Because the regulations for nursing homes are very strict and detailed, nearly all nursing homes receive some "tags" or citations for violations. Thus, just because a nursing home has been cited does not necessarily mean it is a "bad" nursing home. Try to collect as much information as possible to assess the seriousness of any past violations.

Once you have checked the quality record of a nursing home, you should visit the facility. It is a good idea to make both a scheduled visit and at least one unscheduled visit. During the scheduled appointment, you can ask questions of the director of nursing, the facility social worker, or the facility administrator. The unscheduled visit will allow you to judge the typical atmosphere of the home. It is a good idea to pick a time that is typically busy in order to see whether the staffing levels are adequate and how well the staff handles resident requests for assistance. For example, morning is usually a busy time because residents are being assisted with showers and dressing, breakfast, and morning medications. An evening visit may help you assess how the nursing home functions when the administrator and director of nursing have gone home for the day.

A benchmark for evaluating nursing homes that is easy to remember is the "three C's"—compassionate care, cleanliness, and choice. Appearances can be deceiving. An elegantly furnished nursing home may be understaffed or staffed with indifferent personnel. For someone who must now live in a nursing home, compassionate staff will mean much more than color-coordinated furnishings. Likewise, the cleanliness of the facility is more important than fancy furniture. Most seniors would also prefer some flexibility and choice about daily routines, meals, and room furnishings. For example, does the nursing home always offer a few alternative food items in addition to the set menu for the day? Is there choice about shower schedules? May residents watch television late in the evening, or is there a curfew? Respecting and encouraging residents to make choices about what to wear, what to do, and what to eat go a long way toward softening the otherwise institutional atmosphere of a nursing home.

Notes

1. Known officially as a "home equity conversion mortgage," an FHA-insured reverse mortgage is subject to rules found at 24 C.F.R. §§206 *et seq*. The regulations provide that the borrower must pay an initial mortgage insurance premium equal to 2 percent of the maximum amount of the claim and a monthly mortgage insurance premium equal to 0.5 percent per annum on the unpaid balance of the loan (24 C.F.R. §206.105).

2. http://www.aarp.org/money/revmort.

3. See Lawrence A. Frolik and Melissa C. Brown, *Advising the Elderly or Disabled Client* (2008 Supp.), chap. 15: 9.

For More Information

AARP (202-434-AARP)
(http://www.aarp.org)

Find timely discussions about senior housing topics, such as aging in place, house sharing, reverse mortgages, adult day care, age-restricted housing, planned communities, assisted living, CCRCs, and nursing homes, by entering these individual topic phrases into the search engine on the AARP home page.

Eldercare Locator (800-677-1116)
(http://www.eldercare.gov)

Find resources for aging in place in any U.S. community. Links are provided to state and local Area Agencies on Aging and community-based services.

National Hospice Foundation (800-658-8898)
(http://www.hospiceinfo.org)

Find information about hospice care and support services for seniors and their families.

National Long-Term Care Ombudsman Resource Center
(202-332-2275)
(http://www.ltcombudsman.org)

Find state and regional ombudsmen by using the locator search link, as well as general information about residents' rights and current issues in long-term care.

NCCNHR: The National Consumer Voice for Quality Long-Term Care (202-332-2275)
(http://www.nccnhr.org)

Find helpful links, information, and consumer support for improving long-term care practices, programs, and service delivery.

Nursing Home Compare
(http://www.medicare.gov/NHcompare)

Find detailed information about the quality of all nursing homes that are certified to receive Medicare and Medicaid funds.

U.S. Department of Housing and Urban Development (HUD)
(800-333-4636)
(http://www.hud.gov/groups/seniors.cfm)

Find resources for aging in place in your own home or apartment, as well as housing options for seniors who need assistive services.

8

Mental Incapacity, Guardianship, and Conservatorship

Did You Know?

- Without a power of attorney, you may need a guardianship if you lose the ability to make decisions for yourself.
- Guardianship terminates many legal rights and privileges, such as the ability to vote, sign a contract, and make a will.
- A guardian may have the power to make medical decisions, including whether to terminate life support for a mentally incapacitated person.
- With advance planning, no one should need a guardianship.

You may know someone—an elderly parent or relative or perhaps a neighbor—who is no longer able to make decisions about his or her own personal care and finances. This inability to make decisions is likely the result of illness or injury—either dementia resulting from a disease such as Alzheimer's or Parkinson's or a mental impairment caused by a stroke or head injury. If this person has not planned ahead for a substitute decision-maker, there may be no alternative but to seek a guardianship.

This chapter explains what it means to have a guardian appointed for an incapacitated person and what the consequences are for that person's legal rights and privileges. The different types of guardianship are discussed, as are the standards the court uses to decide whether a guardianship is needed and who should serve as the guardian. Finally, the chapter provides an overview of how to obtain a guardianship.

Mental Capacity

The law presumes that every adult has the mental ability, or mental capacity as it is commonly known, to make rational decisions about his or her property and person. Note that the law assumes only that an adult has the ability to make rational decisions; the law does not require a person to make sensible or "good" decisions. Individuals who have the ability to make rational decisions are free to make eccentric, foolish, or even "bad" choices; that is the right of all adults who have mental capacity.

Although the law assumes that all adults have mental capacity, not all do. Some adults suffer from developmental disabilities that cause them to be mentally incapacitated. Other adults who once had mental capacity lose it as a result of injury or illness. These incapacitated persons are in a form of legal limbo, unable to make their own decisions but with no one else who has authority to act for them. Not surprisingly, the law provides a solution for incapacitated individuals.

When an individual lacks the mental capacity to make rational choices, the law permits another person, a substitute decisionmaker, to make legally binding decisions for the incapacitated individual. In the eyes of the law, it is as if the substitute decisionmaker "stands in the shoes" of the mentally incapacitated individual because the decisions of the substitute decisionmaker are treated as if the mentally incapacitated individual made them.

There are two methods of creating a substitute decisionmaker. If a person has planned ahead, then the substitute decisionmakers named in that individual's durable power of attorney and health care advance directives can act if the person later loses capacity (see Chapter 9 for a discussion of durable powers of attorney and health care advance directives). If a person has failed to plan ahead, or the named substitute decisionmakers are not available to act, then a court will have to appoint a guardian.[1]

Guardianship

A state's authority to determine whether an individual is mentally incapacitated and to appoint a guardian comes from the state's general authority to protect the welfare of its citizens. All states have given their courts authority to determine who lacks mental capacity, appoint a guardian, and oversee the acts of the guardian.

Traditionally, courts have viewed guardianship as a protective arrangement for the benefit of the incapacitated person. The view that guardianship is for the good of the incapacitated person often resulted in guardianship laws and standards that did not adequately safeguard the legal rights of vulnerable persons. In the last twenty years, advocates for vulnerable persons have recommended reform of guardianship laws to ensure that protection is provided in a manner that least restricts the rights and privileges of persons with diminished capacity.

Guardianship can indeed provide needed protection for a vulnerable person, but it is also a very intrusive, public intervention. Appointment of a guardian generally terminates the incapacitated person's right to make decisions about his or her own person and property. Furthermore, certain personal rights and privileges cannot be delegated to a substitute decisionmaker and are just lost when an individual is declared legally incapacitated. These include voting rights, driving privileges, the ability to make a will, and decisions about marriage and divorce. Thus, guardianship results in a significant loss of personal freedom and autonomy.

Due to the growing awareness of the intrusive aspects of guardianship, almost every state has now reformed its laws to make the process of obtaining guardianship more protective of the alleged incapacitated person's rights. These reforms include refining the definition of incapacity and creating procedural safeguards such as the right to notice of the hearing, the right to be present at the hearing, and the right to have legal representation. Today's guardianship statutes also require greater judicial supervision of the guardian. As a result of the guardianship reform movement, there are now new and more flexible forms of guardianship, more involvement of lawyers, and more awareness of the need to balance protection of individuals with diminished capacity with their right to autonomy. Although guardianship laws differ, several states have adopted, and many more have modeled their laws on, the Uniform Guardianship and Protective Proceedings Act (8A U.L.A. 429 [2003 and Supp. 2008]).

Guardianship reform has also resulted in more emphasis on individuals planning to avoid guardianship through the use of durable powers of attorney for property management and health care advance directives to guide future medical decisions. The increased use of these documents has significantly reduced the need for guardianship, which can be expensive, time consuming, embarrassing, and possibly contrary to the incapacitated person's wishes. Yet despite the availability of alternatives, most individuals fail to properly plan for incapacity. For them, guardianship is often unavoidable.

Guardianship Terminology

Guardianship is the legal process of providing a substitute decisionmaker for a mentally incapacitated individual. Every state and the District of Columbia has a statute that defines when a person is legally incapacitated and that authorizes courts to conduct guardianship hearings and appoint guardians. There is no federal law of guardianship.

Although "guardian" and "guardianship" are the most common terms for a court-appointed substitute decisionmaker and the arrangement under which that decisionmaker serves, a few states use the terms "conservator" and "conservatorship." In some states, "guardian" refers only to a decision-maker for personal matters, such as health care decisions, whereas the term "conservator" refers to a decisionmaker for property matters, such as investment decisions. In most states, however, the terms "guardian and guardianship" are used to describe the substitute decisionmaker for both person and property.

The incapacitated individual for whom a guardian or conservator has been appointed is often referred to as the "ward," although some states have adopted the term "incapacitated person," with a few states retaining the older term "incompetent." In this chapter, unless otherwise indicated, the terms "guardian" and "guardianship" are used to include the duties of a conservator and the concept of conservatorship. The incapacitated individual for whom a guardian has been appointed is referred to here as the "ward."

For Whom May a Guardian Be Appointed?

State law defines for whom and under what conditions a court can appoint a guardian. Although state laws differ in their definitions of what it means to be incapacitated, the most common description is someone who lacks the ability to make or communicate rational decisions. To determine whether a person is incapacitated, courts consider the individual's behavior and ability to care for essential needs. This functional approach to capacity is a sharp departure from past statutes that often labeled individuals as incompetent merely by virtue of their status, such as "old age."

The goal of functional-based definitions is to narrow the use of guardianship to only those persons who truly lack the mental capability to care for themselves. Just because a person is old, disabled, or mentally ill does not necessarily mean that the person should be considered legally incapacitated. It is how the individual functions, and whether that individual is capable of considering information, making decisions, and appreciating the possible consequences of those decisions, that is important. In short, under modern guardianship laws, courts should order the protection of guardianship only when it is clear that an individual is mentally incapable of caring for his or her own needs.

For Whom May a Conservator Be Appointed?

In some states, the terms "guardian" and "conservator" refer to individuals who serve quite different functions. In those states, guardians are appointed to make decisions about the person of the incapacitated individual, whereas conservators manage the incapacitated or disabled individual's property. Where this distinction is made, a conservator is appointed if for any reason, including severe physical disability, a person is unable to manage or direct the management of his or her property and as a result the property is at risk of being wasted or of being exploited by others. A conservator is often required to manage funds for the support, care, and welfare of the disabled person.

In states that make a distinction between guardianship and conservatorship, the standards for the two usually differ. A lower standard is used for conservatorship—something less than the mental incapacitation required for guardianship. For example, if it can be shown that an elderly person is easily influenced by a manipulative relative to turn over her Social Security funds or pension benefits each month, a conservator may be appointed to manage that individual's money even though she is not truly mentally "incapacitated." In contrast, states that use the term "guardianship" for protective arrangements that cover both person and property usually have a single definition of what it means to be an incapacitated person.

Demonstrating the Need for a Guardian

As a result of guardianship reforms, most state statutes no longer ask why the individual lacks capacity but whether he or she lacks capacity. Nevertheless, the need to identify the cause of incapacity may be important. Many states require a medical explanation for the incapacity as a way of distinguishing true incapacity from mere idiosyncratic behavior that might threaten the individual's health or well-being. For example, consider individuals who choose to participate in "extreme" sports where injury and even death are likely. Although such behavior carries a high probability of personal harm, an adult who chooses to engage in such behavior is not mentally incapacitated if he or she appreciates the possible consequences of the activity and knowingly accepts the risk. Laws that require a medical explanation for incapacity are an attempt to ensure that eccentric but mentally capable persons are not classified as incapacitated.

No matter how a state statute defines incapacity, anyone filing a guardianship petition should be prepared to present expert medical testimony that explains the loss of capacity. Although the burden of proof is on the petitioner, if the alleged incapacitated person believes that a guardianship is unnecessary, he or she should also be prepared to present evidence in rebuttal—that is, evidence that demonstrates his or her capacity to make rational decisions. The standard of proof can vary by state—some require only a "preponderance of the evidence"—in other words, enough evidence to show that it is more likely than not that the person is truly incapacitated. A growing number of states require "clear and convincing evidence" of mental incapacity. This standard requires the petitioner to produce evidence that demonstrates a high probability that the alleged incapacitated individual meets the state's definition of incapacity. The clear and convincing evidence standard is more difficult to meet than the preponderance of the evidence standard, but it is more protective of the alleged incapacitated person's rights and autonomy.

Establishing that an individual lacks mental capacity is only the first step toward obtaining a court-appointed guardian. Just because an individual is incapacitated does not automatically mean that a guardian is needed. If the incapacitated person's needs are being met by other arrangements, such as a durable power of attorney, the court may refuse to approve a guardianship. Again, although it is the petitioner's responsibility to prove the need for guardianship, a substitute decisionmaker who is already acting for the incapacitated person should be prepared to demonstrate that the present arrangement is adequate.

Not all courts, however, are willing to defer to a substitute decisionmaker already acting under a durable power of attorney. The reluctance of some state courts to give priority to a private arrangement for substitute decision-making reflects the concern that agents acting under a durable power of attorney, unlike guardians, are not under the supervision of the court. In theory, unsupervised agents, as compared with court-supervised guardians, can more easily exploit, neglect, or negligently handle the incapacitated person's affairs. However, in actuality, court resources for monitoring guardians are very limited, thus making the distinction between agents and guardians less significant in practice than in theory.[2]

Although state courts vary in their willingness to appoint a guardian, the underlying reality remains that a petitioner for guardianship must demonstrate to the court's satisfaction that a guardianship is truly needed; namely, that the appointment of a guardian would better serve the incapacitated person than existing arrangements. In most states, guardianship is based upon the twin pillars of mental incapacitation (or at least diminished capacity) and an unmet need for services and protection. Absent proof of either of these elements, a court may deny the petition for guardianship.

Types of Guardianship

The type of guardianship granted by a court depends on both the ward's needs and the court's jurisdiction. In order for a guardianship petition to fall under a court's jurisdiction, either the prospective ward or the ward's property, or both, must be located in the state where the court presides. A court can neither grant guardianship over the person of an individual who is not physically present in that state nor grant the guardian authority over property that is physically located in another jurisdiction.

If the alleged incapacitated person resides in the court's state of jurisdiction and has property there, the type of guardianship granted by the court will depend on the incapacitated person's needs and the suitability of the person who wants to be the guardian. Traditionally, there were three types of guardians: guardian of the estate with authority over the ward's property (sometimes referred to as a "conservator"), guardian of the person with authority over personal decisions for the ward, and plenary guardian with authority over both the property and person of the ward.

As a result of guardianship reform, there is now a fourth type of guardianship that operates as a modification of the three traditional types. This newer form of guardianship is known as "limited guardianship." As the name suggests, limited guardianship only grants the guardian power over the ward's person or property to the extent that the individual needs assistance. For example, a limited guardian might control the ward's investments, but the ward may be allowed to retain control over funds to pay for day-to-day expenses. The ward's abilities must be carefully evaluated by the court to determine where to draw the lines of authority between the limited guardian and the ward.

Guardian of the Estate

If the ward needs help with the protection and management of his or her property, the court can create a guardianship of the estate, also known in some states as a conservatorship. A guardian of the estate will usually have the same authority over the property as the owner would have, although there are some limits on a guardian's authority.

Limits on the Guardian of the Estate's Authority. Although the guardian of the estate generally has the right to act as he or she believes best, state law may limit or prohibit certain acts. For example, if the guardian wishes to transfer assets of the ward, state law may (1) permit the guardian to act without prior court approval, (2) require the court to grant authority to transfer such property at the time the guardian is appointed, (3) require the guardian to seek court approval before any transfer, or (4) prohibit the guardian from making a particular transfer. Acts that need prior court approval differ from state to state. Common activities that require prior court approval include selling the ward's real estate and liquidating the ward's investments.

Although a guardian of the estate has no official authority over decisions about the personal care of the ward (such as medical treatment), in reality the guardian's control of the purse strings can have a significant impact on personal decisions. Consider, for example, a situation where two adult children have been appointed as guardians for their mother—one, the guardian of the estate and the other, guardian of the person. The guardian of the person believes her mother should remain at home and be cared for by hired in-home caregivers. The guardian of the estate believes that such care is too expensive and refuses to authorize the payments. A guardian of the estate can also initiate actions that will result in significant lifestyle changes for the ward, such as insisting that the ward's house be sold. It may be necessary to petition the court for removal of a guardian of the estate or a guardian of the person if the two cannot cooperate for the ward's best interests.

Voluntary Conservatorship. In many states, a frail or vulnerable adult may choose to turn over control of assets and financial affairs to a conservator. Because of the voluntary nature of the arrangement, there is no need for incapacity to be proved. Thus, the individual in need of help can receive assistance without the stigma of being found incapacitated and without losing other important legal rights and privileges.

Guardian of the Person

A guardian of the person makes decisions that affect the person of the ward, including decisions about living arrangements and health care matters. State law determines the scope of authority that can be given to a guardian of the person and may prohibit certain acts or require prior court approval for them. For example, although a guardian of the person has the right to determine where the ward will live, the guardian may need prior court approval before moving the ward into a nursing home. Other aspects of the ward's life are considered so personal that no guardian may interfere with them, such as decisions to marry or divorce. No guardian can consent to a marriage, and in most states a guardian cannot initiate divorce proceedings. If the ward's spouse has initiated divorce proceedings, usually the guardian can consent only with prior court approval.

Whether a guardian can consent to mental health care treatment for a ward, even a ward who resides in a mental health treatment facility, varies from state to state. Given that individuals generally cannot be forced to take medication to alleviate the symptoms of mental illness, the guardian, as a substitute decisionmaker, usually cannot commit the ward to such treatment. A guardian of the person normally has the right, however, to make non–mental health care decisions for the ward, such as consenting to medical tests and treatment.

Much more controversial is whether a guardian, without prior court approval, can agree to withhold or terminate life-sustaining treatment. For example, state law varies on whether a guardian of a terminally ill patient may decide to discontinue a feeding tube or a respirator without prior court approval. Increasingly, guardians are permitted to make such decisions without going to court.

Plenary Guardianship

Plenary guardianship, which grants the guardian power to make decisions over both the ward's property and person, is the broadest type of guardianship and allows the guardian to make whatever decisions are necessary for the ward's well-being. Family members who serve as guardians are typically appointed as plenary guardians because they are viewed as well situated to know what the ward needs and how the ward would have made decisions if able. Plenary guardianship, however, can be a double-edged sword.

The plenary guardian has extraordinary power over the life of the ward but is subject to little supervision. Even though this extensive power can result in efficient decisionmaking, it also means that the guardian has a greater opportunity to exploit, neglect, or mistreat the ward. In contrast, where a separate guardian for the property and guardian for the person are appointed, there is a natural check-and-balance on the power of each.

Another challenge of plenary guardianship is finding someone with the ability, time, and desire to undertake the responsibility of acting in all matters for the ward. Although spouses are usually willing to take on such duties, they may be prevented by physical limitations or mental capacity issues. If the spouse cannot act as guardian or there is no spouse, adult children are commonly appointed as guardians. Unfortunately, many adult children do not live near their parents and have difficulties carrying out the duties of a guardian, especially those relating to the ward's property.

Appointing a nonfamily member as guardian is possible if someone is willing to accept that responsibility. If no one is willing to volunteer, professional guardians exist who, for a fee, will assume the role of guardian. Some attorneys are willing to serve as a guardian, as are some geriatric social workers. If the ward has enough income or assets, a bank or other financial institution may be willing to accept appointment as guardian because the ward can afford to pay the costs of the guardianship. Whenever a professional guardian is selected, care must be taken to ensure that the individual or entity is competent, experienced, and honest.

Limited Guardianship

In addition to the three traditional types of guardianship, most courts now have the authority to appoint limited guardians. In the past, individuals were thought of as being either competent or incompetent. Today it is understood that capacity runs along a continuum. In between complete capacity and complete incapacity, individuals may have varying degrees of ability to handle management of their property and persons. For those who are partially incapacitated, the courts can appoint a limited guardian whose powers are tailored to deal with the individual's particular needs. The authority of the guardian is limited in scope so that the ward can be as independent as is possible. For example, a court may appoint a limited guardian who has authority only over the individual's investments, with the individual making all other decisions about his or her life.

The goal of limited guardianship is to permit the ward to retain the maximum degree of independence while giving the ward the assistance he or she needs. Despite the apparent advantages, limited guardianships are not commonly used by courts. They are thought by many to be too time consuming and expensive to be of much practical value. If the ward's condition is one that is likely to deteriorate, opponents of limited guardianship argue that the court will be required to frequently reassess the ward's abilities and adjust the scope of the limited guardian's authority. Without question, evaluating the degree of diminished capacity and crafting a guardianship that least restricts the ward's life take time and money. It is far easier to appoint a traditional plenary guardian.[3]

The costs of limited guardianship aside, they are seldom sought for individuals who still retain some level of capacity because those individuals can most likely still create a durable power of attorney and avoid the courtroom. If they are so incapacitated that they cannot execute a valid power of attorney, then a full guardianship, rather than a limited one, is usually required.

Temporary or Emergency Guardian

A temporary or emergency guardian may be appointed when a quick response is necessary to protect the person or property of the alleged incapacitated person. The terms "temporary guardian" and "emergency guardian" usually have the same meaning. Temporary or emergency guardianships differ from the other types of guardianships. The petitioner does not have to meet all of the normal procedural requirements, and the guardianship is limited in duration. For example, notice requirements are often waived or shorter than for a full guardianship hearing, and the temporary guardianship may be granted without an independent evaluation of the ward's capabilities.

Temporary guardians may be appointed to deal with an immediate crisis, such as the need for a health care decisionmaker for a very sick individual or for facilitation of the discharge of an individual with reduced mental capacity from a hospital. If the patient is too confused to understand the release papers, the hospital or family may need to petition the court for the appointment of a temporary guardian whose authority is limited to signing the necessary discharge papers and moving the patient back home or into a nursing home or an assisted living facility.

Financial emergencies can also require the appointment of a temporary guardian. If an incapacitated person is being financially exploited, a concerned individual can file for temporary guardianship to stop the exploitation by taking control of the ward's assets and initiating civil or criminal proceedings against the party committing the exploitation.

Although there are fewer procedural formalities required for a temporary guardianship proceeding, the court must still find that the alleged incapacitated person meets the statutory definition of incapacity. If not, the petition for temporary guardianship will be denied. Courts will not approve a temporary guardianship merely as a convenience to the petitioner or as a means of avoiding the procedural requirements of a regular guardianship. Even where a temporary or emergency guardian is appointed, the court may conclude after a full hearing for permanent guardianship that the alleged incapacitated person does not need a guardian or that the need for assistance has passed.

Guardianship Procedures

The Petition

Guardianship is initiated by the filing of a petition that requests the court to find that the alleged incapacitated person is indeed incapacitated and in need of a guardian. In almost every state, any competent adult can file a guardianship petition, but usually only those concerned about the alleged incapacitated person's property or welfare are likely to do so. Institutions, such as hospitals, may file petitions because they need an individual who can sign consent, admission, or discharge forms on behalf of an incapacitated patient. Occasionally, bank officers or trustees may file a guardianship petition if they believe that a customer can no longer handle his or her financial affairs. The person who files the petition is known as the petitioner. Typically, the petitioner is, but need not be, the person nominated in the petition to serve as the guardian.

General Content Requirements. The contents of a guardianship petition depend on applicable state law and local court rules. As a result of guardianship reform, many states now have detailed requirements for what the petition must include. Usually, the petition must name the alleged incapacitated person; the cause, nature, and extent of the incapacity; and the type of guardianship sought (of the person or property, limited or plenary). The alleged incapacitated person's address and a description of his or her living arrangements (e.g., whether the person lives alone, with relatives, or in an institution such as an assisted living facility) are usually also required. The petition must explain the reason a guardianship is needed and how appointment of a guardian would benefit the alleged incapacitated person. The state may also require an explanation as to why no less-restrictive arrangement is appropriate. A petition that fails to meet all of the state or local requirements may be dismissed. Normally, an attorney is hired to draft and file the petition.

Nomination of the Guardian. State law or local court rules require the petition to contain the name and address of the proposed guardian. The requirement of naming a guardian can pose difficulties. If no family member or close friend is willing to serve as guardian, the petitioner may have to consider a professional guardian. Professional guardians, however, may be too costly and may not be available in all communities. Some states finance public guardians, but they are usually overworked and may be limited to acting as guardian only for the poor. The shortage of persons to serve as substitute decisionmakers is a growing problem in our aging society.

Where to File the Petition. Guardianship petitions are usually heard by the probate court (a court that hears matters of wills and estates). The proper place to file a petition is the county in which the incapacitated person lives or in which he or she happens to be physically present. A petition for guardianship of the estate can be filed in a county where the incapacitated person owns property.

Changing the Residence of the Ward. If the ward moves to a different state after a guardianship is established, a petition must be filed in the new state to have the guardian's authority recognized there or to have a new guardianship established in that state. State law varies as to whether the new state will accept the guardian's authority over the ward. Some states allow reappointment of a guardian merely upon proof of the original appointment in the prior state. Other states have laws permitting the transfer of a guardianship.[4]

Petitions Involving Property Located in a Different State. Often wards own vacation or rental property in a state other than the one in which they live and hold most of their property. If it is necessary to sell or rent that property for the benefit of the ward, a petition for guardianship over that property will have to be filed in the state where the property is located. The law of the state where the property is located may permit its court to rely upon a finding of incapacity in another state, or it may require a hearing to determine whether a guardian should be appointed. In any event, the authority of the guardian of the estate will be limited to dealing with the ward's property located in that state.

Notice

By statute, almost all states require that the alleged incapacitated person be given notice of the filing of the petition and the hearing date. Most states also require notice to be given to a variety of other persons, including the incapacitated person's spouse, family members, creditors, and heirs at law. Some states require notice to the person or entity that has physical custody of the alleged incapacitated person, such as a nursing home. States differ as to the amount of notice, but at least seven to fourteen days before the hearing date is common.

The Hearing

Before a guardian can be appointed, a judicial hearing must occur for the purpose of deciding whether the individual is mentally incapacitated and, if so, to what extent. To inform the court's decision, many states require a medical or psychological examination of the alleged incapacitated person. Incapacitation usually must be proved by clear and convincing evidence, which means that the judge or jury must be persuaded by the evidence that the claim of incapacitation is highly probable.

If the individual is found to meet the state's definition of incapacity, the court will have to decide whether a guardianship is in the best interests of the incapacitated individual. The petitioner must provide evidence that the needs of the mentally incapacitated person are not currently being met and that a guardian is needed. Based on this evidence, the court must determine what kind of guardianship will best serve the incapacitated person's needs—a guardianship for property, for the person, or both (plenary)—and whether that guardianship should be limited. Finally, the court must determine who should be named as the guardian or guardians. All of these decisions, of course, require evidentiary support. The purpose of the hearing is to consider that evidence.

Presence of the Alleged Incapacitated Person. The hearing requirements vary from state to state and even from court to court. Nevertheless, some standards are common. All states permit the alleged incapacitated person to attend the hearing; a few require his or her presence. Even if state law permits the court to hold the hearing without the alleged incapacitated person, most courts are reluctant to do so. To ensure the incapacitated person's presence, courts now commonly hold the hearing at the individual's residence, even in a hospital if necessary.

Right to a Jury. Though many states permit the alleged incapacitated person to request a trial by jury, most prefer an experienced judge to rule on the issue of incapacity. In some hotly contested guardianship hearings, however, counsel for the alleged incapacitated person may prefer that a jury, rather than a judge, determine the client's mental capacity in the belief that the jury may be more sympathetic to an older individual who is attempting to avoid the stigma and loss of autonomy that accompany guardianship. If the jury decides that the individual is incapacitated, the judge will then determine whether a guardian is appropriate and who will be named guardian.

Court Visitors. In some states, courts have the authority to seek information about the alleged incapacitated person before the formal hearing. Where permitted, the court can appoint a visitor who interviews the alleged incapacitated person, determines whether he or she should be present at the hearing, investigates his or her living conditions and financial well-being, and reports back to the court, perhaps with a recommendation as to what the court should do. The visitor may also interview the petitioner for information about why the petition was filed and talk to the proposed guardian to see if he or she is capable of carrying out the responsibilities of the position. Even though the final decision as to the alleged incapacitated person's mental capacity and need for a guardian is made by the court, the court visitor's findings can be critical in that determination.

Right to Legal Counsel. Because of the potential loss of autonomy for the ward, most, but not all, states require that the alleged incapacitated person be represented by legal counsel. The lawyer will be paid out of the assets of the ward whenever possible. If the alleged incapacitated person cannot afford a lawyer, the state provides one and will bear the cost. Counsel representing an alleged incapacitated person must pursue the client's wishes, even if the apparently incapacitated client wishes to resist guardianship.

Guardian ad litem. A guardian *ad litem*, though typically an attorney, is not the alleged incapacitated person's legal counsel. A guardian *ad litem* is an officer of the court who is expected to inform the alleged incapacitated person about the meaning of the guardianship hearing and to listen to that individual's concerns. The guardian *ad litem*, however, is not required to advocate for what the alleged incapacitated person wants, but rather is expected to make an independent decision about what would be in that individual's best interest and so inform the court. Therefore, because of their different obligations, the counsel to the alleged incapacitated person and the guardian *ad litem* should not be the same person.

Selection of the Guardian
If the individual is found to be incapacitated and in need of assistance, a guardian must be appointed. If more than one person or entity wishes to serve as guardian, the court is supposed to select the candidate who will best serve the needs of the ward. Several considerations influence how the court decides among competing candidates for guardian.

Guardian Nominated by the Petitioner. Given that the court does not have the power to force anyone to be a guardian, the court's choice is limited to those who are willing to serve. More often than not the court will appoint the individual or entity nominated in the petition unless there is a good reason not to do so. If no one is available to serve as guardian, the court may have the power to appoint a guardian who will be paid by the state.

Petitioners should identify the potential guardian before filing the petition. There are probably potential petitioners who do not file petitions because they are unable to locate a guardian. Many people do not want to serve as guardian because of the time it takes or because they are reluctant to assume the role of making critical life choices for another individual. Guardians of the estate are somewhat easier to find because the duties, although time consuming, are more manageable as they do not usually have the emotional burdens associated with being a guardian of the person.

Nomination of Guardian by the Ward. Some wards will have previously nominated a guardian, possibly in a durable power of attorney or a health care advance directive. In most states, if the ward has previously nominated someone for guardian, that individual, if qualified and willing, must be named as guardian, although an alternative individual can be named if the court finds good cause for doing so. If the ward has only modestly diminished capacity, the court may inquire as to whom the ward might wish to be named guardian. If the ward's choice is appropriate, the court will name that person as guardian.

Statutory Priorities. Some state statutes list possible guardians in order of their priority, usually beginning with the person nominated by the ward, followed by a spouse, children, and other relatives. A qualified individual with the highest priority is supposed to be named as guardian. If there are persons with equal priority, the court is directed to select the one best qualified to be the guardian. The court can pass over a person with higher priority to select someone with lower or no priority only for a good reason. The statutes also often exclude as candidates for guardian individuals with conflicts of interest, such as employees of the nursing home where the ward resides.

Even though circumstances may at times require the use of a professional guardian, courts prefer family members because they assume that family members, who are bound by ties of love and devotion, will perform better than a professional motivated only by professional standards and compensation. In contrast, even if a family member is willing to serve as guardian, the court may instead appoint a professional guardian if the court finds that to do so is in the best interest of the ward. Usually, the reason for a professional appointment is family discord—either discord between competing would-be guardians or discord between the ward and the proposed guardian. Conflicts of interest can also cause a court to reject a family member.

In recent years, state laws have been liberalized to permit nonprofit entities to serve as guardians. These social service entities are usually paid from the funds of the incapacitated person or by the county or state. They often serve as guardians for "friendless" individuals who do not have a willing or able family member, relative, or friend, and who do not have enough assets to afford the cost of a professional or institutional guardian such as a bank.

Several states have created public guardians to act as the guardian of last resort when no private individual or entity is available. Public guardians are agencies, offices, or public officials whose job it is to act as guardian of the estate or of the person. The cost of the public guardian is paid from the funds of the ward if there are sufficient assets, and if not, the state bears the cost. In a few states, public guardians are actively involved in the day-to-day details of the incapacitated person's life. In other states, because of a large caseload, the public guardian acts only to make major decisions in health care and living arrangements. Even when a public guardian exists, however, that office usually lacks the resources to assist all eligible elderly wards.

Costs of Guardianship

Guardianship is costly. Filing a petition requires hiring an attorney, paying for medical or other professional examinations, paying the fee of a court visitor or guardian *ad litem*, compensating witnesses such as physicians for their time, and perhaps hiring a social worker to prepare a care plan. If the case is appealed, additional legal costs will be incurred.

The costs of guardianship are borne by the ward subject to court approval. The attorney who represents the alleged incapacitated person is entitled to payment so long as the attorney rendered valuable services that were consistent with the alleged incapacitated person's wishes. Even the attorney for the petitioner is paid from the ward's funds provided that the petition for guardianship is successful. However, if the petition is denied, the petitioner is usually responsible for all fees and costs of litigation associated with pursuing the petition.

If the ward's funds are inadequate to pay the fee of his or her attorney, state law may provide for payment by the state or county. Unfortunately, the statutes often set a very low rate of fees, which tends to discourage attorneys from accepting appointment as counsel for alleged incapacitated individuals. Recently, some courts have requested that the legislature take steps to increase attorney fees to a more reasonable level.

Once appointed, the guardian is entitled to a fee for his or her services as well as reimbursement for out-of-pocket expenses. Often family members will decline any fee, though they are still entitled to any out-of-pocket expenses that they incur. Naturally, professional guardians expect to be paid, usually receiving an hourly fee, although if they act as guardian of the estate, they may be paid an annual fee equal to a percentage of the value of the ward's assets. Nonprofit entities that serve as guardian are usually paid a flat amount for each guardianship. Note that no fee can be paid to any guardian without prior court approval. If the court believes the requested fee is too high in comparison to the services performed by the guardian, the court will reduce the fee to a more appropriate amount.

Supervision of the Guardian

The actions of guardians are subject to the control and supervision of the court. Most states require annual reports to be made by the guardian. Reports by the guardian to the court are intended to promote guardian accountability for meeting the ward's needs. The guardian is expected to confer with the ward prior to making major decisions and then to make decisions consistent with the ward's expressed desires. If the ward cannot communicate, the guardian is expected to act in a manner consistent with the ward's preferences as they existed before the onset of the incapacity. If the incapacitated person never expressed a preference, the guardian is expected to act as a reasonable person would under the same or similar circumstances.

Initially, the guardian of the estate will be required to inventory the incapacitated person's assets and file an accounting with the court. Thereafter, the guardian will typically be required to provide an annual accounting with the court, although sometimes the court will insist upon more frequent reports. Usually, the guardian will have to account for all income received and expenses paid, and upon the termination of the guardian's term, the guardian will have to turn over all the assets of the ward. Mistakes, misuse, or intentional misconduct by the guardian can result in the guardian's personal liability for the ward's losses as well as penalties assessed by the supervising court.

Guardians of the person must also report to the court in most states. In many states, the guardian of the person must make an initial status report about the ward. The guardian may also be required to provide the court with a care plan and indicate how that plan will meet the ward's needs. The court can also require the guardian to report after a period of time about the ward's progress under the plan. In a report by the guardian of the person, the primary requirement is to describe any changes in the ward's mental and physical condition, note any unmet needs of the ward, and advise the court whether the guardianship should be continued or whether the powers of the guardian should be modified.

Guardians who fail to carry out their obligations may be removed by the supervising court or ordered to act in a more appropriate manner. Generally, state law permits any interested person, including the incapacitated person, to petition the court for the purpose of making it aware of guardian misconduct.

Termination of the Guardianship

A guardianship ends at the death of the incapacitated person. In the event of the death, mental incapacity, or resignation of the guardian, however, the guardianship does not terminate. Instead, the court appoints a successor guardian. Normally, no guardian will be permitted to resign unless there is an available successor guardian, because the incapacitated person cannot be left without a substitute decisionmaker.

If the incapacitated person regains capacity, the guardianship should be terminated. Generally, the incapacitated person must petition the court and request that it terminate the guardianship. Whereas in the past the burden was on the ward to prove that he or she had regained capacity, many states have reformed their guardianship statutes so that the burden of proof is now on those who want to continue the guardianship. If the ward petitions the court to end the guardianship, those who want it to continue must persuade the court that the ward is still incapacitated and that the continuation of the guardianship would be in his or her best interest.

Notes

1. For an in-depth analysis of the use of a durable power of attorney as an alternative to guardianship, see Linda S. Whitton, "Durable Powers as an Alternative to Guardianship: Lessons We Have Learned," *Stetson Law Review* 37 (2007): 7.

2. For an up-to-date overview of court guardianship monitoring practices in the various states, see Naomi Karp and Erica F. Wood, "Guardianship Monitoring: A National Survey of Court Practices," *Stetson Law Review* 37 (2007): 143.

3. For a discussion of the difficulties in getting greater use of limited guardianship, see Lawrence A. Frolik, "Promoting Judicial Acceptance and Use of Limited Guardianship," *Stetson Law Review* 31 (2002): 735.

4. The Uniform Law Commission approved in 2007 the Uniform Adult Guardianship and Protective Proceedings Jurisdiction Act (8A U.L.A. 1 [Supp. 2008]), the purpose of which is to resolve multistate guardianship jurisdiction disputes and to facilitate transfers of guardianship between jurisdictions where appropriate. For a list of states that have adopted the act, see the Uniform Law Commission website at http://www.nccusl.org.

For More Information

National Guardianship Association (877-326-5992)
(http://www.guardianship.org)

Find links to publications and other resources for family guardians.

9

Substitute Decisionmaking for Health Care and Property

Did You Know?

- If you lose capacity and have no substitute decisionmaker, you will likely need a court-appointed guardian.
- To avoid guardianship, you need a substitute decisionmaker for both health care decisions and decisions about your property and finances.
- You can name different substitute decisionmakers to handle health care and property decisions.
- You should carefully choose your health care agent because he or she may make life and death decisions for you when you can no longer decide for yourself.
- You should carefully choose your agent for property decisions because he or she will likely have access to all of your property, including your money.

All adults need to plan for management of their health care and property in the event they later lose the ability to make and carry out their own decisions. No one wants a guardianship, which involves public exposure, expense, and loss of control. Fortunately, for those who plan ahead, alternatives exist that can eliminate the need for guardianship.

Alternatives to guardianship allow you to appoint an individual or institution to act as your substitute decisionmaker or "agent." Because courts are generally not involved in these alternatives, they are less costly than guardianship. However, because these alternatives are not court supervised, the risk exists that your agent may take advantage of you. You should there-fore choose an agent whom you wholeheartedly trust—someone who will act according to your expectations even if you cannot monitor what the agent is doing.

In order to prevent the need for guardianship, you must make sure that a substitute decisionmaking plan is in place for both health care decisions and property management. The name of the document for appointing a health care agent varies from state to state. The person appointed may be called your health care "proxy," "representative," or "agent," depending on the language used in your particular state's statute. Every state also has a power of attorney statute that allows you to give someone else authority to make your property and financial decisions. The person appointed to act for you under a power of attorney is called your "agent" or "attorney-in-fact."

You do not have to choose the same person to serve as the agent for both health care and property decisions. For example, Betty, a widow, feels that her daughter would be the best suited among her children to make decisions about her finances and property because the daughter is a certified public accountant. Although her daughter lives in another state, Betty is confident that her financial affairs can be handled long distance through online ac-count management and telephone communication. With respect to substi-tute decisionmaking for health care, Betty chooses to make her son her health care agent because he lives in the same town and would likely be available in the event of an emergency.

Depending on the complexity of your property matters, you may decide to name an institution, such as a bank or trust company, rather than an indi-vidual, to serve as your agent. Whereas it is customary for family-member agents to serve without compensation, institutions charge a fee that is typi-cally a percentage of the value of the property they are managing. Thus, an institutional agent may not be a good choice for seniors with only modest property and financial reserves.

The following discussion explains in greater detail how you can create a substitute decisionmaking plan for your health care and property manage-ment. Although a health care proxy and a durable power of attorney for property management are the primary tools for avoiding guardianship, there are other legal arrangements, such as a trust, joint account, or Social Security Representative Payeeship, that can serve a substitute decisionmak-ing function. These are also discussed.

Substitute Decisionmaking for Health Care

Creating a substitute decisionmaking plan for health care involves (1) stat-ing in advance *what* kind of treatment you would want if you could no longer make those decisions for yourself and (2) selecting *whom* you would want to make decisions on your behalf. The first type of planning is sometimes called *directed* decisionmaking because you direct now—while you have capacity—what you would want later if you no longer have the ability to make decisions. The second type of planning is referred to as *delegated* decisionmaking because you delegate to someone else the authority to make decisions for you if later you cannot make the decisions for yourself.

In most states, the document used to direct what you would want if you later lose capacity is called a living will. The document that is used to delegate health care decisionmaking authority to someone else is usually called a health care proxy or power of attorney. The term "health care advance directive" is frequently used to include both living wills and health care proxies.

So long as you still have the mental capacity to make your own decisions, your wishes trump the opinions of anyone you have appointed as your health care agent. Likewise, if you change your mind about the choices stated in your living will or whom you want to serve as your health care agent, you can revoke your health care advance directives and create new ones.

Directed Health Care Decisionmaking

There are two basic types of health care documents that can be used to direct your medical treatment if you later lose the ability to make your own decisions. One is a directive that you can prepare without a physician's assistance, commonly called a living will. The other is a physician's order based on your wishes. Depending on state law, physician orders may include Do Not Resuscitate (DNR) orders, Out-of-Hospital Do Not Resuscitate orders, and Physician Orders for Life Sustaining Treatment (POLST).

Living Wills. Under all state laws today, you can sign a health care directive—commonly called a living will—that specifies whether you would want life sustaining treatment if you have a terminal illness or injury. Life sustaining treatment may include ventilators or respirators to help you breathe, cardiopulmonary resuscitation if your heart stops, and tube feedings to supply water and nutrition if you cannot eat or drink. The U.S. Supreme Court has recognized the right of all competent citizens to accept or decline medical treatment as well as the right of each state to set its own standard of evidentiary proof for whether an individual has made a choice about life sustaining treatment (*Cruzan v. Mo. Dep't. of Health*, 497 U.S. 261 [1990]). The much publicized cases of Nancy Cruzan (*id.*) and Terri Schiavo (*In re Guardianship of Schiavo*, 916 So.2d 814 [Fla. Dist. Ct. App. 2005]) illustrate the difficulties that can arise if a person has not clearly indicated in writing what his or her wishes are with respect to life sustaining treatment.

There is no right or wrong decision when it comes to a health care directive about life sustaining treatment. Each person should decide, based upon individual values and beliefs, what course of treatment would be preferable in a terminal situation. Whether you choose to accept or decline life sustaining treatment, you should discuss this decision with your health care providers and your family so that they will understand what you want if you can no longer participate in the decisionmaking process.

Under federal law, hospitals must ask patients whether they have health care advance directives, and if a patient does not, hospitals must offer the patient an opportunity to create them (Patient Self-Determination Act of 1990, Pub. L. No. 101-508, §§4206, 4751, 104 Stat. 1388). However, some physicians and religiously affiliated hospitals may not be willing to follow a health care advance directive that requests the discontinuation or the withholding of certain life sustaining procedures such as tube feedings. It is important to ask whether your physician or hospital has any policies that conflict with your wishes. If there is a conflict, you may need to seek care from providers whose policies are consistent with your preferences and values.

DNRs, Out-of-Hospital DNRs, and POLST. For patients who have terminal or serious, progressive chronic conditions, there are additional directed decisionmaking tools that may be important. These include DNRs, Out-of Hospital DNRs, and POLST. Unlike a living will, which is created and signed by the patient, DNRs, Out-of-Hospital DNRs, and POLST protocols are directives about life sustaining treatments that are prepared by a physician after talking with the patient or the patient's health care agent.

The most common of these physician orders, the DNR, specifies that a patient should not be resuscitated in the event that the patient's heart stops. Because such orders are effective only for patients residing in a hospital or skilled nursing facility, an increasing number of states have enacted Out-of-Hospital DNR statutes that permit patients with terminal or serious, chronic conditions to have portable DNR orders. Such patients wear an Out-of-Hospital DNR identification tag to avoid resuscitation by emergency medical services if they happen to suffer cardiac arrest while outside of a hospital or skilled nursing facility.

Some states recognize a POLST protocol. POLST laws are aimed at ensuring that the wishes of those who have advanced, chronic progressive illnesses can be put in portable medical orders. These orders are more comprehensive than DNRs and cover, in addition to cardiopulmonary resuscitation, other medical treatment decisions such as hospitalization, tube feedings, antibiotics, and ventilation to assist breathing.

Delegated Health Care Decisionmaking
Whereas a living will and advance physician orders are important tools for stating today what you would want if you were terminally ill or in the end stages of a progressive illness, these directed decisionmaking tools do not cover all of the circumstances in which medical decisions might be needed on your behalf. For example, what if you were unconscious as the result of an automobile accident and could not participate in decisions about your

care? Or what if you were conscious but unable to communicate due to the effects of a stroke? Because there are many nonterminal medical scenarios in which you might need care but lack the ability to participate in treatment decisions, it is important that you consider whom you would want to make those decisions for you.

If you do not select someone to act as your health care decisionmaker, most states have laws that allow certain family members (usually your spouse, adult children, and adult siblings) to give medical consent for you. However, these laws are at best a fallback method for substitute decision-making. You may not have relatives that qualify under the statute, or you may prefer that someone other than a relative act for you. Difficulties can also arise if the family members qualified by statute do not agree about your care. Most statutes do not give an order of priority among possible family decisionmakers. If qualified family members cannot agree about your treatment options, a guardianship may be necessary to resolve the dispute.

To avoid the problems that can result from reliance on family consent laws, it is usually better to appoint a substitute health care decisionmaker. The name for this person varies by state, as does the name of the document for appointing the person. Common names include health care representative, health care proxy, and health care agent. No matter what the name, this individual should be someone you trust and someone who is willing to carry out your wishes if you are unable to participate in your own treatment decisions.

The best way to ensure that your wishes will be followed is to discuss your values and preferences with your health care agent. Although incapacity and the possibility of serious or terminal illness are not pleasant topics of conversation, a candid discussion about these topics is the only way your health care agent can know your wishes. Knowing what you want will also reduce some of the stress for your agent if such decisions later need to be made.

How to Make Your Plan for Substitute Health Care Decisions Work

Make Your Plan Known. Your health care decisionmaking plan will be effective only if your doctors and agents are aware of it. Discuss your wishes and values with your doctors, agents, and family members to ensure that they understand what you want and are willing to make decisions that are consistent with your wishes. If you have different agents for health care and financial decisions, make certain that both agents fully understand what you want. Even though your health care agent may have the authority to make your medical care decisions, the cooperation of your financial agent is necessary to pay for such care. Likewise, family members who do not have actual decisionmaking authority for you should be informed of your plan so that you can reduce the likelihood that they will later challenge the actions of your agents. Keep a card in your wallet that identifies the contact information for your health care agent and any successor agents.

Sign Multiple "Originals" of Your Documents. Although in most states your health care providers are allowed to rely on a copy of your living will and health care proxy or power of attorney, it is a good idea to sign several "originals" when your documents are prepared. Your agent and any successor agents should be given documents that contain an original signature, and you should keep a reserve set somewhere that is easily accessible in the event of an emergency.

Be Aware of Different State Law Requirements. The legal requirements for preparing a valid living will and health care proxy vary from state to state. Usually, state law requires that health care advance directives be signed and witnessed. Some state laws require two witnesses. Whether advance directives prepared in one state will be honored in another state varies state to state. Consequently, if you regularly live in more than one state, or plan to receive health care in another state, it is a good idea to prepare health care advance directives that meet both states' requirements. Another option is to prepare a separate set of documents for each state.

Substitute Decisionmaking for Property and Financial Management

The most common and cost-effective way to create a substitute decisionmaking plan for property and financial management is the durable power of attorney. All states have power of attorney laws that permit adults with decisionmaking capacity to give another person the authority to deal with their property and finances. The person who grants such authority is called the "principal." The person who receives authority from the principal is called the "agent" or "attorney-in-fact." All states allow these powers of attorney to be durable—that is, they continue to be effective even if the principal later loses decisionmaking capacity. Thus, a durable power of attorney is the most common technique for avoiding guardianship.

In addition to the durable power of attorney, there are other legal devices that can be used for limited substitute decisionmaking. In most instances, they are used in addition to a power of attorney rather than in its place. These include a trust, jointly held financial accounts, and a representative payeeship for management of a person's Social Security benefits.

Durable Power of Attorney
A durable power of attorney is a document that gives another person—known as your agent—authority to act on your behalf with respect to your property and money. In this arrangement you are known as the principal. If the power

of attorney is *durable*, your agent will continue to have authority to act on your behalf even if you lose the ability to make and carry out your own decisions. Most people want their power of attorney to be durable so that they can avoid the need for guardianship if they later become incapacitated.[1]

In some states, all powers of attorney are durable unless stated otherwise in the document. In others, the power of attorney has to contain language that indicates the principal's desire that it remain valid even if the principal later loses capacity. A power of attorney can also be written so that it becomes effective only if the principal loses capacity. This is known as a springing power of attorney.

Whether you should choose an immediately effective power of attorney or a springing one depends on your objectives. If you are interested in giving an agent authority *only* as a precaution to avoid guardianship, then a springing power might be preferable. However, if you want your agent to be able to take care of your property and financial matters when you are out of town, or perhaps too ill to run errands, then the convenience of an immediately effective power of attorney may best suit your circumstances.

Regardless of when you want your power of attorney to become effective, the most important choice you must make is deciding who should serve as your agent. A power of attorney is no better than the trustworthiness of the agent acting under it. In order for your power of attorney to provide effective protection against the need for guardianship, you should also name a successor agent who can act for you if your first agent is no longer willing or able to act.

Almost as important as your choice of agent is the decision about how much authority to give to your agent. Although broad authority is usually a good idea if your goal is avoiding guardianship, you should exercise caution when giving your agent authority that could put your property at risk or impact your estate plan. For example, an agent with authority to make gifts, to create or revoke trusts, or to create or change beneficiary designations and survivorship interests could completely undermine your estate plan.

You may also want to consider whether your initial agent and successor agent should each have the same degree of authority. For example, you might feel comfortable giving your spouse unlimited authority to make gifts or to change beneficiary designations but would not want to see such authority in the hands of one of your adult children. The understanding that you and your spouse have with respect to gift making priorities among your children and grandchildren may not be shared by an adult child who sees sibling fairness issues differently.

In general, an agent is viewed as a fiduciary and is expected to act in the best interest of the principal. This means that an agent cannot use the principal's property for his or her own benefit unless authorized by the power of attorney. Some states have detailed provisions that describe an agent's duties. In states without such provisions, the courts rely on the common law of agency, which is based on case law decisions about the conduct of principals and agents.

In most states, an agent has either a common law or statutory duty to keep track of any dealings with the principal's property and to account for those transactions if requested by the principal, a court, or a representative of the deceased principal's estate. A principal can also include a provision in a power of attorney that requires the agent to make periodic accountings to a third person. Such a provision may operate as a safeguard on the agent's activities or as a way to prevent suspicions from arising where one child is selected over others to serve as the agent.

Although the law does not require a power of attorney to be prepared by a lawyer, it is advisable to seek out a lawyer's advice so that your power of attorney can be adjusted to fit your needs and objectives. Nearly one-half the states have an optional statutory form that can be used to create a power of attorney. Care should be taken to make sure that you satisfy the requirements for your state.

Some states require that the power of attorney be notarized. Others require one or two witnesses. Still others may require only the principal's signature. If your power of attorney may be used in a real estate transaction, notarization is advisable because it is required by county recorders' offices before documents such as deeds can be placed in the public record. Because powers of attorney are governed by state law, it may be necessary to do more than one power of attorney if you own property in more than one state. However, an increasing number of states are honoring out-of-state powers of attorney if they are valid under the law where they were created.

Advantages of a Power of Attorney. Compared with guardianship or a trust, a power of attorney is the most cost-effective and flexible form of substitute decisionmaking for property. There is no need for the principal to be officially declared incapacitated, and the transactions with respect to the principal's property can remain private. If the principal still has capacity and changes his or her mind about the choice of agent or scope of authority, the principal can simply revoke the power of attorney and create a new one.

Unlike a trust arrangement, which is effective only to deal with property titled in the trust, a power of attorney can authorize the agent to pursue personal entitlements and claims on the principal's behalf, such as those arising under Social Security, Medicare, and Medicaid laws, or under contracts and dealings with other persons. Another advantage of the power of attorney is that title to the principal's property remains in the principal, as opposed to trust assets, which have to be retitled in the name of the trust.

Disadvantages of a Power of Attorney. The greatest disadvantage of a power of attorney is that it is an unsupervised arrangement and susceptible to abuse. The very attributes that make it desirable—the privacy and flexibility with which the principal's affairs can be handled—make it potentially dangerous if placed in untrustworthy hands. Theoretically, it is a trustee's accountability to the terms of the trust document and a guardian's account-ability to the court that protect vulnerable persons in those arrangements. In reality, however, these arrangements likely offer little more protection than the power of attorney. Court systems often lack the resources to monitor the activities of guardians, and a family trustee may have no one to whom the trustee must account other than the now incapacitated beneficiary. On balance, if care is taken in the selection of the agent and the scope of au-thority delegated to the agent, a power of attorney remains the best all-purpose tool for substitute decisionmaking.

Revocable (Living) Trust

Revocable trusts—also referred to as "living" trusts—are a common way to avoid probate (i.e., property passing under a will at your death) and provide incapacity planning for substitute management of property and finances. Property in a trust does not pass under your will at death because the prop-erty is titled in the name of the trust rather than in your name. A person called a trustee is responsible for managing the trust assets according to the instruc-tions in the trust document. You can name yourself as the initial trustee, but a successor trustee should also be named to take over trust management re-sponsibilities if you later lose capacity or no longer wish to manage the assets.

Consider the example of Sarah, an 85-year-old widow, who transferred her certificates of deposit, savings account, and a brokerage account into a revocable trust. Sarah named herself as the sole trustee and her 60-year-old daughter, Doris, as successor trustee. Two years after the trust was estab-lished, Sarah was diagnosed with early stage dementia and no longer felt comfortable managing the trust. She simply resigned as trustee, thus permit-ting Doris to take over as successor trustee. Doris now manages the funds in the trust and uses them to pay Sarah's living expenses.

Even though most people name spouses and children as successor or co-trustees, any adult with decisionmaking capacity can serve in that role. Indi-viduals with considerable wealth often name professional trust companies to act as trustee. Institutional trustees charge a management fee based on the value of the trust and thus are not a good choice for persons with only mod-est assets.

No matter what the value of the property to be placed in trust, most peo-ple seek the assistance of a lawyer in creating the trust. The trust instrument sets out all of the terms of the trust, which can be as varied and creative as you like. You may also need assistance changing the titles on property that will be transferred to the trust, such as real estate, bank and brokerage ac-counts, and automobiles.

A trust creates a fiduciary relationship between the trustee, who has title to the property, and the beneficiary, who is the person who receives benefits from the trust. As a fiduciary, the trustee must follow the instructions in the trust document and act in good faith and the best interest of the beneficiary. Usually, the person who creates a revocable trust—called the settlor—is also a beneficiary of the trust during the settlor's lifetime. Thus, it is possible for the original owner of the property to wear three hats—settlor, trustee, and beneficiary during his or her lifetime.

The settlor of a revocable trust may amend or revoke it at any time so long as the settlor has mental capacity. The settlor can replace a trustee or change who will serve as successor trustee. The settlor can also change the beneficiaries. If the settlor becomes incapacitated, the trust becomes irrevocable for as long as the incapacity continues unless the settlor has given revocation authority to someone else. At the settlor's death, the trust continues until the time specified in the trust instrument for it to terminate. When that date is reached, which is often after all of the settlor's debts and estate taxes have been paid, the trust assets are distributed according to the instructions in the trust instrument. Because the assets do not pass through probate, the revocable trust serves as a will substitute as well as an alternative to guardianship.

Advantages of a Revocable Trust. One advantage of a revocable trust is that the property subject to the terms of the trust is clearly identified, as are the duties of the trustee. For those who can afford a professional trustee, the quality of the substitute property and financial management may be higher than under a less formal power of attorney arrangement. Furthermore, financial institutions are often more comfortable dealing with trustees than agents under powers of attorney.

A trust may also provide greater protection for your wishes should you later become incapacitated. You may make your expectations for property and financial management very explicit in the trustee's instructions. For example, if you have the resources to pay for in-home care and you are concerned that family members may move you to institutional care once you become incapacitated, your trust can be created to authorize only payment for in-home care. This directive must be respected, even if the arrangement is more expensive than nursing home care. Expenditures that might otherwise be considered imprudent—such as requiring the trustee to pay for a private room in a nursing home—will be permitted if the trust instrument authorizes them.

Disadvantages of a Revocable Trust. A revocable trust is the most expensive and complicated method of avoiding guardianship. Legal fees are incurred when the trust is created and increase with the trust's complexity. The cost of a revocable trust includes the expense of changing the title to all of the assets that must be transferred to the trust. Professional trustees charge an annual fee for their services, and accounting fees may also be incurred depending on the scope of the trust's activities.

A trust will not avoid the necessity of probate proceedings if the settlor fails to transfer all of her or his property to the trust. This risk is particularly high with respect to items that are obtained after the creation of the trust. Likewise, a revocable trust does not provide any income or estate tax savings for the settlor. The income of the trust is taxed to the settlor regardless of whether it is actually distributed to the settlor. And although the trust assets do not pass through probate, the assets are included in the deceased settlor's estate for purposes of state inheritance tax and federal estate tax.

Jointly Held Financial Account

Jointly held financial accounts can serve a variety of purposes. You may want to add the name of another person to your bank account for the sake of convenience only—that is, to permit the other person to conduct financial transactions on your behalf, but without transferring any ownership interest to that person. Or you may wish to give that person part ownership of the account and survivorship rights in the money held in the account. If you give a "true joint tenancy" interest in your bank or brokerage account to another person, that person is treated as receiving a present share of the account as well as survivorship rights in the total account.

Unfortunately, many financial institutions do not distinguish between a "convenience account" and a "true joint tenancy account" on the forms and signature cards used to open the account. The primary reason for this is that financial institutions want to avoid liability with respect to withdrawals made from accounts held in more than one name. Typically, any named owner on a jointly held account may access all of the funds in the account. Thus, a jointly held account is one way of providing for substitute management of account assets if one of the account holders later loses decision-making capacity. However, as the following examples illustrate, a power of attorney may be a better method of establishing a substitute decisionmaker if the sole purpose of a joint account is convenience.

Consider the example of Bob and Mary, both in their 80s and suffering from chronic health conditions that make it difficult for them to run errands. Bob and Mary have a joint-tenancy bank account that includes rights of survivorship. In part, they chose this type of account so that when one of them dies the survivor will have all of the account assets without the necessity of going through probate. Because it is physically difficult for them to go to the bank, Bob and Mary decide to add Tom, Bob's son from a former marriage, to the account so that he can help them with banking errands. This arrangement works well until Tom withdraws half of the money after Bob's death, claiming that it is his through rights of survivorship. Another problem can occur if Tom, who was added for convenience purposes only, has creditors who want to attach assets in the account to satisfy Tom's debts.

A few states have enacted laws that require banks to provide customers with the option of different account titles that distinguish true joint tenancy accounts from convenience accounts. Where such laws do not exist, courts generally permit the persons who contributed the money to the account (or their heirs) to offer proof that the other named person on the account was authorized for convenience purposes only.

Although it is possible to obtain a court ruling on the true intent of an account held in more than one name, lawsuits are time consuming and expensive. If a true joint tenancy is not intended, care should be taken to assure that the account title accurately reflects the convenience nature of the arrangement. If it is not possible to open an appropriately titled account, then use of a power of attorney to give the substitute decisionmaker authority over the account (but no appearance of ownership) better achieves the intended objective.

Social Security Representative Payeeship

If a senior who receives Social Security or Supplemental Security Income benefits needs assistance managing these payments, a representative payee can be appointed by the Social Security Administration (42 U.S.C. §§405[j], 1007, 1383[a]). A payee may be appointed either because the beneficiary wants assistance or because Social Security believes that the beneficiary needs assistance. If a family member or friend is not available to serve as payee, Social Security may appoint a qualified organization.

All children and legally incapacitated adults who receive benefits are required to have representative payees. Even if an incapacitated person has an agent who has been appointed to serve under a power of attorney, Social Security requires that the incapacitated person also have a representative payee. The agent under the power of attorney may apply to become the representative payee.

To become a representative payee, a person must submit an application at the local Social Security office and supply proof of identity. With limited exceptions, Social Security requires a face-to-face interview with the representative payee applicant. Individual representative payees may not charge a fee for their services, but they may be reimbursed for out-of-pocket expenses. Qualified organization payees must be authorized in writing by Social Security to charge a fee for representative payee services.

Representative payees must use payments solely for the benefit of the beneficiary, such as paying for food, shelter, clothes, and medical care. Any benefits not spent on past bills or current needs must be saved for the beneficiary's future needs. The representative payee must keep a record of all payments received and how they were spent or saved. The payee must also complete a Representative Payee Report, which Social Security sends out once a year.

A beneficiary who suspects that the payee has misused benefits should contact Social Security so that an investigation can be conducted. If Social Security was negligent in permitting misuse of the benefits, Social Security must repay the funds to the beneficiary. If Social Security was not at fault, the beneficiary is responsible for reclaiming the misused benefits from the representative payee.

If a beneficiary believes that he or she no longer needs a representative payee, the beneficiary may request that the representative payeeship be terminated, but the beneficiary must convince Social Security that the need for the arrangement no longer exists. Social Security may request a physician's statement that the beneficiary's condition has improved and that he or she is now capable of managing benefit payments.

How to Make Your Plan for Substitute Property and Financial Management Work

Choose Your Substitute Decisionmaker Carefully. Whether you are considering a power of attorney, trust, joint bank account, or representative payeeship, any substitute decisionmaking arrangement is only as good as the substitute decisionmaker. You should choose someone who is not only trustworthy but who will respect your wishes and carry them out even if you no longer have the ability to monitor what is happening. If you are using a power of attorney or trust, you should also choose a trustworthy successor agent or trustee so that your substitute decisionmaking plan does not fall apart if something happens to your original substitute decisionmaker.

Discuss Your Expectations. You should have a candid discussion with anyone who will have authority as your substitute decisionmaker and explain how you want your property and money handled. For example, under what circumstances would you want your property sold or given away? If you are using a power of attorney, do you want your agent to continue a pattern of gift giving or family maintenance if you lose the capacity to do so? Do you expect your agent to serve without compensation?

Carefully Consider How Much Authority to Give Your Agent. Although it is important to give your agent broad enough authority to avoid a guardianship, there are certain powers that may be particularly risky in the hands of an agent. These include the power to make or revoke a trust, to give a gift of your property, and to create or change beneficiary designations and survivorship interests. Such powers may be appropriate in the hands of your initial agent, but not a successor. For example, Bob may want his wife, Carol, to have such powers, but not his daughter, Anne, who is named as his successor agent.

Communicate Your Expectations to Family Members Who Might Challenge Your Plan. Although there is no sure defense against family members who might try to upend your substitute decisionmaking plan, candidly discussing your plan and choice of agent may make it more difficult for them to launch an attack. Creating a written record of your expectations and instructions for your substitute decisionmaker may also make it more difficult for others to argue that you wanted something (or someone) else.

Note

1. For a general discussion of the use and benefits of durable powers as an alternative to guardianship, see Linda S. Whitton, "Durable Powers as an Alternative to Guardianship: Lessons We Have Learned," *Stetson Law Review* 37 (2007): 7.

For More Information

ABA Commission on Law and Aging Consumer's Tool Kit for Health Care Advance Planning
(http://www.abanet.org/aging/toolkit/)

Find worksheets and resources that will help you consider your values and choices when preparing health care advance directives as well as suggestions about how to choose and communicate with your substitute decisionmaker.

Social Security Administration Internet Support for Representative Payees
(http://www.ssa.gov/payee/index.htm)

Find information for representative payees as well as information for beneficiaries who have a representative payee. A link is also provided for filing a representative payee accounting online.

10

Elder Abuse, Neglect, and Exploitation

Did You Know?

- Most abusers are people close to the victim—usually family members or caregivers.
- Most communities have agencies and programs to help abuse victims.
- Keeping vulnerable seniors connected to their communities with home visits and phone calls can reduce or prevent elder abuse.
- Your identity will be protected if you report suspected elder abuse.

"Elder abuse," as that term is used in the law, applies to more than just physical and psychological harm; it also includes neglect and financial exploitation. Many factors make it difficult to track how often elder abuse, neglect, and exploitation occur. Even though there is no central reporting system, the National Committee for the Prevention of Elder Abuse estimates that 4–6 percent of all elderly are abused. In the past, elder abuse was frequently hidden or dismissed as uncommon, but today government and social service agencies acknowledge that elder abuse, neglect, and exploitation occur frequently. This chapter looks at the nature and causes of elder abuse, the circumstances in which it often occurs, and what you can do if you, or someone you know, are victimized or in danger of becoming a victim.

What Are Abuse, Neglect, and Exploitation?

Abuse, neglect, and exploitation form the trio of what is usually just called elder abuse. Abuse can be conduct or statements that injure or threaten the physical or psychological well-being of an older person. Even onetime physical assaults, if harmful enough, are considered elder abuse. Inappropriate restraint of a person is a form of physical abuse. For example, a caregiver who ties an older person in bed for hours so that he or she will not get up unassisted and fall is committing an act of elder abuse. Nonconsensual sexual contact of any kind is also a form of physical abuse.

Psychological abuse, even though it may leave no physical injury, is no less serious than physical abuse. It can range from threatening to abandon the older person, or to put him in a nursing home, to threatening physical force if the person does not cooperate in daily tasks such as eating, bathing, and taking medication. Even repeated insults and shouting are a form of psychological abuse because they undermine the victim's sense of self-worth and security.

"Exploitation" is the term frequently used to describe financial abuse—that is, the misuse or theft of another person's property and money. Blatant forms of financial abuse include using the victim's ATM card without permission to withdraw money, or using the victim's power of attorney to steal the victim's property or money from bank accounts. More subtle forms of financial exploitation can occur when the abuser has close and frequent contact with the victim—such as where a relative caregiver shares the same home with the victim. The caregiver may be able to slowly siphon off the older person's assets. This can be accomplished by taking more than a fair share of that person's monthly retirement or Social Security benefits for the common household expenses or by spending the older person's money for the benefit of other family members. Abusive family members who pay for expensive vacations, houses, or automobiles with the elderly relative's money may justify the expenditures on the grounds that the money will be theirs someday anyway, or that the elderly victim is also benefiting from the expenditures.

Abusive acts often contain elements that are physical, psychological, and financial. For example, a family member may bring an elderly relative to his home for a "visit" and then seek permanent guardianship over that relative, arguing that he or she is no longer able to handle personal care and financial decisions. Using guardianship as a means to control the older person and his or her assets can be a form of legal "kidnapping" when that individual is not in a psychological position to freely object to the arrangement. Threats of nursing home placement or emotional abandonment may pressure the older person into going along with the arrangement. Domineering family members have also been known to cut off communication between elderly relatives and other family members or friends. The increasing frequency of adult children fighting over their parents and their parents' assets has prompted some elder advocates to call these guardianships "will contests while the person is still alive."

Unlike acts of physical, psychological, and financial abuse, which involve intentional threats or conduct, neglect is a failure to act that puts the older victim at risk. For example, it is elder neglect when a caregiver fails to provide essential medicine, food, or shelter to an older person. Liability for neglect is based on a legal "duty" to act. That duty is usually based on a contract when the neglect occurs in a nursing home or at the hands of someone hired to provide home care.

Neglect by family members who have volunteered to care for an elderly person at home may be more difficult to prove. No family member, with the exception of a spouse, has a duty to provide care to another adult. However, once that responsibility has been accepted and the vulnerable person has become dependent on that care, most states recognize that the volunteer caregiver has a duty to continue that care or to seek out an alternative caregiver. For example, Adam begins to provide daily help to his 88-year-old grandfather, Grant, who lives next door and must use a wheelchair. Having let Grant become dependent on his care, Adam cannot simply go on an extended vacation without making some provision for Grant's care while he is gone.

Most state statutes that deal with protection of vulnerable older persons also include "self-neglect" as a basis for protective legal intervention. This intervention may take the form of voluntary acceptance of protective services such as home-delivered meals or housekeeping assistance or involuntary measures such as guardianship. Appropriate protective intervention depends on the degree of self-neglect and the ability of the vulnerable adult to make rational decisions. Although self-neglect is often listed as a type of elder abuse that will trigger protective intervention, it is really not abuse in the technical sense. Rather, self-neglect is a descriptive term for a person's inability to care for herself or to make appropriate arrangements for such care.

Where Does Elder Abuse Occur?

Elder abuse occurs both in institutional settings, such as nursing homes, assisted living facilities, and board and care homes, and in noninstitutional settings, such as the victim's home or the home of a caregiver. Although the impact on the victim is essentially the same in either setting, where the abuse occurs is relevant to answering questions about how to effectively help victims and how to prevent the abuse from happening again. Whether in an institutional or noninstitutional setting, abuse occurs more frequently to seniors who are dependent and isolated.

Institutional Settings

Abuse in an institutional setting is usually perpetrated by individual employees. Physically abusive acts may include hitting uncooperative residents and using excessive physical restraints or drugs to keep residents contained and less demanding of staff time. Sexual assault is another form of physical abuse that can occur in institutional settings.

Neglect in an institutional setting usually takes the form of inadequate attention to resident needs, such as not responding to call buttons, providing substandard care, or failing to provide a decent emotional atmosphere of safety and concern for the older person's well-being. Signs of neglect in nursing homes range from residents who have infected bedsores due to lack of proper repositioning in their beds to residents who suffer severe weight loss and kidney failure from dehydration and inadequate assistance with eating.

Although residents are discouraged from keeping cash in their rooms, financial exploitation still occurs in an institutional setting. Financial abuse includes not only theft of whatever petty cash the resident might keep in the room, but also theft of residents' personal belongings, such as jewelry, radios, and televisions. As a result, the freedom to enjoy one's jewelry and other valuables can be compromised by the need to protect property from theft while residents are sleeping or out of their rooms for meals and activities.

Abuse and neglect are more common in institutions that serve the poor because such institutions often cannot afford to hire quality employees or to provide decent care. Undertrained, overworked, and poorly supervised employees too often lash out at the residents. Financially stressed institutions may cut corners on the amount of staff and other services in order to meet budget. The isolation and dependency of the residents and their lack of housing alternatives leave them no choice but to endure these unsatisfactory living conditions.

Even institutions that serve the middle class frequently have too few staff, pay low wages, and provide inadequate training. One of the primary reasons for this is inadequate public funding for those residents who have run out of money to pay for their own care. Medicaid, a hybrid program financed by both the federal and state governments, is the sole source of payment for a majority of nursing home residents. Unfortunately, the Medicaid reimbursement rates pay only about 70 percent of the actual cost of such residents' care, leaving nursing homes to find creative ways to balance their budgets.

Noninstitutional Settings

Abuse in a noninstitutional setting usually happens at the hands of a caregiver, often a family member. Because incidents of slapping or yelling at the victim often occur in the privacy of the victim's home or home of the caregiver, the victim's friends or other family members may be unaware that it is happening. Some victims put up with the abuse for fear they will lose the caregiver or that the caregiver—often an adult child—will get into trouble with the law. Other victims are too isolated or too physically or mentally incapacitated to seek help.

Some abuse occurs when caregivers fail to understand the older person's medical needs. For example, Judy is caring for her elderly aunt May, who suffers from diabetes. Judy does not understand the importance of diet in controlling Aunt May's diabetes and so fails to provide a proper diet or to monitor what Aunt May eats. Other abuse is just very negligent caregiving. It may range from failing to seek medical attention soon enough for the older person to more intentional abuse, such as leaving bedridden persons to lie in their own waste or refusing to feed them by hand because it is "too much work."

Financial exploitation by caregivers is fairly common and difficult to uncover. Some caregivers enter into the relationship specifically to financially exploit the victim. Often the victim is not even aware of the exploitation. For example, when the caregiver lives with the victim, it is easy to commingle funds and use the older person's money for the caregiver's support. The elderly victim may be lonely or depressed and believe that flattering attention by a caregiver or a "new best friend" is genuine. In such circumstances, the victim can be manipulated into making gifts or giving the abuser access to the victim's bank accounts and other property.

Causes of Abuse, Neglect, and Exploitation

Some who abuse the elderly are persons who have the specific, bad intent to exploit or injure their victims. They select the elderly as victims because they are available, vulnerable, and less likely to report the abuse. Others— usually family members—believe that they are entitled to use the victim's property and money as "payment" for caregiving or as part of the inheritance that will eventually be theirs. In other cases, caregivers simply become so frustrated with their duties and so angry with the older person that they lash out from the fatigue of caring for someone who may be uncooperative or even physically and verbally abusive to the caregiver. To be sure, the stress of caregiving can lead to despair, anger, and resentment, but abuse is never a proper response. Caregivers should seek available social services and other forms of support that will lessen their burden.

Studies have found that some abuse is revenge motivated—adult children retaliating against their older parents for abuse committed against them as children. Other abusers consider violence a normal and acceptable way of responding to someone who is uncooperative or burdensome. Many abusers suffer from alcohol or drug dependency and financially exploit the elder person to obtain money for their addiction. Caregivers who are financially dependent upon the older person may subconsciously resent their dependency and respond by abusing, neglecting, or exploiting the older person. For others, abuse is a way of gaining control and satisfying an emotional need to dominate the victim.

Solutions

Area Agencies on Aging and Adult Protective Services
Every state has enacted laws designed to protect the elderly from abuse, neglect, and exploitation. The federal government contributes limited funds to

states to help combat the problem. Federal grants are made to each state's agency on aging, which in turn provides money to local Area Agencies on Aging (AAAs). The state agency on aging serves as a general coordinator of all services and programs related to the assistance of elderly people within the state. The local AAAs supervise the actual delivery of services, usually at the county level.

The Older Americans Act Amendments of 1987 require state agencies on aging to assess the need for elder abuse prevention services and to create a state plan to prevent elder abuse within the state (Pub. L. No. 100-175, §144, 101 Stat. 926, 948-50 [1987]). Unfortunately, the federal funding to prevent elder abuse has never been sufficient, which explains in part why the problem is still so prevalent. Despite the lack of adequate funding, states have enacted adult protective services statutes as a means of establishing a comprehensive response to the problem of elder abuse. The statutes define elder abuse, provide ways to uncover it, establish the guidelines for protective interventions, and create punishments for the abusers.

All the statutes define elder abuse as physical harm. Some include the infliction of mental anguish or psychological injury, although that is sometimes limited to psychological abuse that is severe enough to require medical attention. A few states recognize unreasonable confinement as elder abuse, as well as neglect that rises to the level of a failure to provide for basic needs, including food, shelter, and care for physical and mental health. Self-neglect can be the basis for an investigation if the individual's personal safety is an issue. Financial exploitation is also included as abuse and is generally defined as the illegal or improper use of an elderly individual's resources or property for the benefit of the exploiter or another.

Many of the adult protective services laws require reporting of suspected abuse by professionals, such as health care personnel, social service providers, law enforcement officers, social workers, physicians, and nurses. To encourage nonmandatory reporting, all states guarantee to protect the identity of abuse reporters, although a few states permit limited disclosure of the reporter's identity under special circumstances. All states' statutes provide for some sort of initial investigation when a report of alleged abuse is received. The investigation will be carried out by a state or county agency. A few states require that the local law enforcement agency investigate elder abuse complaints.

After an investigation is completed, or if the older person requests assistance, the protective services agency is supposed to take the steps necessary to terminate the abuse and to meet the older individual's care needs. Usually, protective services include several types of assistance, such as a visiting nurse or home health aid, Meals-on-Wheels, light housekeeping, and legal assistance if necessary. The older person who is believed to be at risk for abuse, neglect, or exploitation must voluntarily accept assistance. If the person does not agree and adult protective services believes that the person is no longer capable of engaging in self-care or making rational decisions about needed care, adult protective services has authority to seek a temporary court order for emergency protective intervention and, when necessary, involuntary guardianship over the person.

Self-neglect often triggers services that the individual may not want. For example, Elaine, age 85, is found in poor condition living in her home, with a dozen or more cats, rotted food and trash all over the house, and no heat. Under many state adult protective services statutes, a state could force its way into the home, remove the animals, and either force Elaine to take care of herself or move her into a facility with supportive services, such as a nursing home.

The involvement of adult protective services can also lead to help for overstressed caregivers who may be well intentioned but who have snapped under the pressure of their caregiving responsibilities. If investigation reveals that the alleged abuser is generally a good caregiver but in need of support and a break, adult protective services may be able to arrange counseling and education for the caregiver as well as regular respite care for the vulnerable elder. Such services provide the caregiver with emotional support as well as periodic relief from caregiving so that the caregiver can attend to his or her own needs.

Criminal and Civil Law Remedies

Most elder abuse is also a crime under various state laws, including laws that criminalize assault and battery, theft, and extortion. In addition, a number of states have enacted statutes that specifically criminalize abuse of the elderly. Unfortunately, in many cases the abused older person will not report the crime out of a sense of loyalty if the abuser is a family member or caregiver or out of fear of retaliation by the abuser. Even if the abuse is reported, the criminal justice system may not respond quickly enough to protect the older person.

Another avenue for relief is a civil suit asking for a restraining or protective order against the abuser. Every state has special restraining orders and protective orders that can be invoked in the case of intrafamily abuse. These statutes, generally referred to as Domestic Violence Acts, permit the victim to obtain a court order forbidding contact between the abuser and the victim and requiring the abuser to leave the victim's household. Unfortunately, some of these statutes can be used only against a spouse. Even a protective order is not a guarantee that the violence or abuse will stop. If the abuser is also the older person's live-in caregiver, the older person may have no alternative other than moving to a nursing home for needed care. A surprising number of elderly would rather endure abusive or neglectful care than move into a nursing home.

Special Solutions for Abuse in an Institutional Setting

If abuse occurs in an institutional setting, there are several state offices whose responsibility it is to investigate complaints and find solutions. The local long-term care ombudsman is responsible for investigating reports of abuse in nursing homes and other residential care facilities (see Chapter 7 for more information about the Long-Term Care Ombudsman program). Although the long-term care ombudsman does not have direct authority to bring civil or criminal penalties against the nursing home or the abusive employee, the ombudsman often works with the nursing home to address and correct abuse problems. In very serious situations, including those involving a pattern of abuse, the ombudsman may assist the state agency that supervises nursing homes (often the state Department of Health or the state Department of Family and Social Services) and the state attorney general's office to pursue civil fines and criminal charges against abusers and the facilities in which abuse has occurred.

The victim, or someone who suspects that a resident has been victimized, may also make a complaint directly to the state regulatory agency for nursing homes or the state attorney general's office. State attorney general's offices have Medicaid fraud and control units that are required to investigate and prosecute patient fraud, abuse, and neglect in facilities that participate in Medicaid.

Community Programs

In addition to government offices that have a responsibility for investigating and addressing elder abuse, many communities have developed cooperative partnerships among seniors, law enforcement, and social service agencies for the purpose of preventing and redressing elder abuse. One such partnership is called Triad. The Triad concept was developed through the collaboration of AARP, the International Association of Chiefs of Police, and the National Sheriffs' Association. Each Triad is formed at the community level and comprises senior citizens, law enforcement agencies, and community groups that provide elder support and protection services.

Triads sponsor both educational programs and assistance in the community to help seniors avoid becoming the victims of elder abuse. Examples of such programs include the following:

- programs on how to avoid criminal victimization
- information on the latest fraud schemes and scams
- guidelines for dealing with telephone solicitations and door-to-door salespeople
- home security information and inspections
- Adopt-a-Senior visits for shut-ins
- safe shopping day programs that provide senior transportation to local grocers

- safe walks programs that arrange transportation to safe locations where seniors can enjoy weekly walking and exercise
- telephone reassurance programs

The success of these and other community-based programs has demonstrated that greater public awareness about the elder abuse problem, education of seniors, and services that keep seniors connected to their communities are essential components in preventing and reducing the incidence of elder abuse.

For More Information

AARP (202-434-AARP)
(http://www.aarp.org)

Find information about how communities can develop programs to fight fraud and abuse.

Eldercare Locator (800-677-1116)
(http://www.eldercare.gov)

Find information about local programs and services, including home-delivered meals, adult day care, caregiver support services, and legal assistance.

National Association of Triads (NATI) (800-424-7827)
(http://www.nationaltriad.org)

Find advice and technical assistance for local Triads.

National Domestic Violence Hotline (800-799-SAFE)
(http://www.ndvh.org)

Find local domestic violence shelters, other emergency shelters, legal aid programs, and social service programs.

National Committee for the Prevention of Elder Abuse
(http://www.preventelderabuse.org)

Find information and links to resources for elder abuse victims as well as for community groups and professionals who would like to improve programs and services for the prevention of crime and abuse against elders.

Index

About the Authors

Lawrence A. Frolik is Professor of Law at the University of Pittsburgh School of Law and an adjunct professor of law for the University of Miami School of Law LL.M. program in estate planning. He was one of the original academic creators of elder law as a scholarly discipline. A prolific author, in addition to his book, *Advising the Elderly or Disabled Client*, he has authored a dozen other books, including *Residence Options for Older or Disabled Clients*, *Elder Law in a Nutshell*, and the casebooks, *Elder Law: Cases and Materials*, and *Law of Employee Pensions and Employee Benefits*.

He is an elected fellow of the National Academy of Elder Law Attorneys, an academic member of NAELA's Certified Advanced Practitioners, and an academic member of the Special Needs Alliance. He is the past chair of the Pennsylvania Bar Association Elder Law Section, and he served as a policy advisor to the Executive Council of the Pennsylvania AARP. He now serves as a fellow of the TIAA-CREF Academic Advisory Board and as a trustee of the Achieva Family Pooled Trust. In 1995, he was a congressional appointed delegate to the White House Conference on Aging.

Linda S. Whitton, Professor of Law at Valparaiso University School of Law, is the Reporter for the Uniform Power of Attorney Act. She is a commissioner of the American Bar Association Commission on Law and Aging, an ABA representative to the National Conference of Lawyers and Corporate Fiduciaries, and a fellow of the American College of Trust and Estate Counsel. She is a past council member of the American Bar Association Section of Real Property, Trust and Estate Law and a past chair of the Association of American Law Schools Section on Aging and the Law. Professor Whitton teaches courses in elder law and property and frequently speaks and publishes on a variety of elder law topics.